T0192577

Real-World Evidence in Drug Development and Evaluation

Chapman & Hall/CRC Biostatistics Series

Series Editors

Shein-Chung Chow, Duke University School of Medicine, USA
Byron Jones, Novartis Pharma AG, Switzerland
Jen-pei Liu, National Taiwan University, Taiwan
Karl E. Peace, Georgia Southern University, USA
Bruce W. Turnbull, Cornell University, USA

Recently Published Titles

Artificial Intelligence for Drug Development, Precision Medicine, and Healthcare
Mark Chang

Bayesian Methods in Pharmaceutical Research
Emmanuel Lesaffre, Gianluca Baio, Bruno Boulanger

Biomarker Analysis in Clinical Trials with R
Nusrat Rabbee

Interface between Regulation and Statistics in Drug Development
Demissie Alemayehu, Birol Emir, Michael Gaffney

Innovative Methods for Rare Disease Drug Development
Shein-Chung Chow

Medical Risk Prediction Models: With Ties to Machine Learning
Thomas A Gerds, Michael W. Kattan

Real-World Evidence in Drug Development and Evaluation
Harry Yang, Binbing Yu

Cure Models: Methods, Applications, and Implementation
Yingwei Peng, Binbing Yu

Bayesian Analysis of Infectious Diseases
COVID-19 and Beyond
Lyle D. Broemeling

For more information about this series, please visit: https://www.routledge.com/Chapman--Hall-CRC-Biostatistics-Series/book-series/CHBIOSTATIS

Real-World Evidence in Drug Development and Evaluation

Authored by

HARRY YANG AND BINBING YU

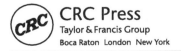

CRC Press
Taylor & Francis Group
Boca Raton London New York

CRC Press is an imprint of the
Taylor & Francis Group, an **informa** business

A CHAPMAN & HALL BOOK

CRC Press
Boca Raton and London
First edition published 2021
by CRC Press
6000 Broken Sound Parkway NW, Suite 300, Boca Raton, FL 33487-2742

and by CRC Press
2 Park Square, Milton Park, Abingdon, Oxon, OX14 4RN

ISBN: 9780367026219 (hbk)
ISBN: 9780429398674 (ebk)

Typeset in Palatino
by KnowledgeWorks Global Ltd.

Contents

Preface

Real-world evidence (RWE) has long been used by regulatory agencies to monitor long-term safety and rare adverse events of marketed drug products. However, it was not until recently that stakeholders in healthcare began embracing RWE as a key driver of outcomes- and value-based strategy in the drug development life cycle. Owing to the advances in digital technologies such as cloud data storage and advanced analytics, including artificial intelligence (AI) and machine learning, real-world data (RWD), collected from disparate sources, have become more connected and effectively interrogated for insights. The new laws, regulations, and growing demand for pharmaceutical companies to demonstrate values of their products to healthcare stakeholders have given the drug developers added incentive to develop comprehensive RWE strategies and capabilities. The recent shift of the drug development paradigm toward a more personalized healthcare and value-based coverage and payment policies has further fueled the use of RWE.

RWE is generated from settings other than traditional clinical trials and may be derived from a variety of sources, such as electronic health records, administrative and claims data, product and disease registries, and patient-generated data including in-home use settings or wearable devices. As evidenced by many successful applications, RWE has proven to be transformative in all aspects of drug research and development (R&D) and commercialization.

In early drug discovery, RWE can help researchers understand patient profiles, disease burden and prevalence, and effectiveness of the standard of care. Coupled with genomic data, RWE may create an opportunity to uncover biomarkers leading to more targeted drug development strategies for clinical development. RWD and RWE can be used to improve trial design operation, including study feasibility, site selection, and patient recruitment. More importantly, RWD can be used to guide innovative trial design such as single-arm trials augmented with a synthetic control arm derived from RWD or pragmatic study to generate evidence of comparative effectiveness. RWE that goes beyond the outcomes from the traditional randomized controlled trials plays a critical role in regulatory assessments concerning label expansion, coverage and payor decision, optimization of drug pricing, and drug supply chain and inventory management.

RWE has disrupted the way new medicines are developed. However, to realize the full potential and deliver the promise of RWE, it is imperative to have not only quality RWD but also the ability to extract insights from complex and heterogeneous data sets. Equally important is the clarity of regulatory policies regarding the use of RWE for registrational purposes. In the published literature, a wide range of applications of RWE and use cases have been discussed, and opportunities and challenges expounded. Despite these publications, there is no single book systematically covering the latest developments in the field.

This book discusses the latest advances in RWD and RWE for drug development and evaluation. The contributors for this book are experienced pharmaceutical practitioners, providing a broad array of RWE perspectives, opportunities, challenges, and solutions. Chapter 1 is an introductory chapter that discusses the evolving role of RWE in the drug development process. Drawing from the published literature and use cases, it highlights the potential opportunities and challenges of RWE applications in transforming drug R&D and commercialization. Chapter 2 expands on the utility and constraints related to RWD and RWE from the author's review of the latest developments together with personal perspectives on the topic that are additionally informed by the author's own research. It concludes with cautions and recommendations related to standards of quality assurance in RWD and the evidence generated from such data in drug development. Chapter 3 describes how to use RWD from a population-based cancer registry to evaluate trends and burdens of cancer. It covers several statistical methods such as micro-linked map and joinpoint model for the analysis and presentation of cancer statistics. Also included is an example of supplementing the clinical trial data with RWD for better extrapolation of survival. Chapter 4 provides an overview of how to adopt external control using RWD and historical control in clinical development. The concepts of synthetic and historical controls are illustrated through several examples regarding the use of RWE to aid drug approval and label expansion. Bayesian methods for evaluating drug safety using RWE are discussed in Chapter 5. Of note is a demonstration of using the Bayesian method to assess the effect of an unobserved confounder based on RWD. Chapter 6 covers the value-based agreements in drug pricing and illustrates how to use RWE for coverage and payment decisions. It also discusses the trends, case studies, and guidance regarding the use of RWE by payers and health technology assessment (HTA) agencies. Chapter 7 reviews the commonly used strategies for inferring causal relationships from observational data using propensity score adjustment. The method is illustrated through an RWD example of trauma care system evaluation. Chapter 8 gives an introduction to AI and machine learning in drug development. Special attention is given to the use of deep learning analyzing electronic health records to predict clinical outcomes.

We would like to thank John Kimmel, executive editor of Taylor & Francis, for providing us the opportunity to work on this book. We are deeply grateful to Deepak Khatry for his expert review and editorial assistance. The editors of the book also wish to express their gratitude to the contributors of the book. Last, the views expressed in this book are not necessarily the views of the authors' respective companies.

Harry Yang
Binbing Yu
Gaithersburg, Maryland

1

Using Real-World Evidence to Transform Drug Development: Opportunities and Challenges

Harry Yang

1.1 Introduction

In recent years there has been a growing interest in using real-world evidence (RWE) to support drug development, regulatory review, and healthcare decision-making. RWE, gleaned from real-world data (RWD), provides useful insights into disease prevalence, innovative trial design, comparative effectiveness and safety of treatment, and health economic value. Coupled with evidence from randomized controlled trials (RCTs), RWE enables drug developers, regulators, and healthcare providers to make more informed decisions. RWE has been at the forefront of pharmaceutical innovations, disrupting the way evidence is generated in the value chain of drug R&D and commercialization. The use of RWE is further powered by the new governmental policies and laws such as the 21st Century Cures Act in the United States and Conditional Approval (Martinalbo et al. 2016) and Adaptive Pathways in Europe (EMA 2016a,b). Leveraging RWE in regulatory decision is a key priority for many regulatory agencies. In the recently released U.S. Food and Drug Administration (FDA) guidance (FDA 2018a), it is stated that under the right conditions, data derived from real-world sources can be used to support regulatory decisions. When extracted from well-designed studies and appropriate analysis, RWE may constitute valid scientific evidence to support the early approval of a drug product, label change, or expansion. In this chapter we present the unprecedented opportunities and challenges of applying RWD and RWE in drug development and evaluation.

1.2 Traditional Drug Development Paradigm

1.2.1 Drug Development Progress

Drug development is a complex, lengthy, and resource-intensive process. Figure 1.1 presents a diagram of drug development.

The process commences with drug discovery. Scientists utilize many technologies such as synthetic chemistry and genomic sequencing to uncover targets that are causes of diseases. When a lead new molecular entity (NME) is identified, it is advanced to a pre-clinical development stage where the NME is tested both in vitro in cells and in vivo in various animal species to determine its safety and efficacy. This is followed by the clinical phase of product development, which typically follows a well-established paradigm, with the primary aim of generating evidence of drug safety and efficacy in support of marketing approval by regulatory authorities. It consists of three phases, Phase I, II, and III trials, with a focus on clinical pharmacology and early safety, efficacy evaluation in targeted patient populations, and confirmation of drug's safety and efficacy, respectively. Potentially, Phase IV studies, often termed post-approval trials, may be required after marketing approval. It is aimed at gaining better understanding of either potential long-term adverse effects or rare adverse events associated with the product. This post-marketing evaluation again draws insights from clinical studies in controlled settings. Clinical trials are often carried out utilizing a mechanism in which

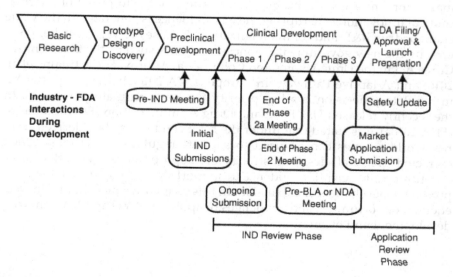

FIGURE 1.1
Drug development process. Adopted from FDA website.

subjects in treatment group(s) or a control group are randomly assigned, and usually referred to as RCTs. Randomization is used to rule out the effects of potential confounding factors and ensure comparable patients across the groups (Barton 2000). Patients in the studies are closely followed to ensure treatment adherence. Additionally, individuals including the medical monitors from sponsors, patients, and investigators are blinded about the patient treatment, and the way data are analyzed is pre-specified. Together, these measures ensure internal validity of the study design and conclusions.

1.2.2 Limitations of Traditional Randomized Controlled Trials

Use of RCTs for demonstrating drug safety and efficacy has been the gold standard for assessing a drug's safety and efficacy. The evidence generation process of an RCT is consistent with regulatory expectations. However, there are several drawbacks concerning the RCT methodology. First, the outcomes from RCTs may lack external validity as RCTs are often conducted under strictly controlled experimental conditions that are different from routine clinical practice. Consequently, RCTs often provide an estimate of the efficacy of the drug rather than the true measure of effectiveness in the real world (Black et al. 1996), resulting in a gap between the efficacy demonstrated in the clinical trials and effectiveness of the drug in real-world use. Factors that contribute to the gap include patient adherence, age, comorbidities, concomitant medications, and so forth. Because of these variations, findings from RCTs may not always translate into the performance of the product in the practical setting. Second, due to rising medical costs, healthcare decision-making by payers has increasingly relied on the balance of cost and benefit of a new treatment. However, despite the demand for demonstration of the value of medical products to justify payment, traditional RCTs offer little information because of the gaps between efficacy-effectiveness. The situation worsens for drug products that are approved based on single-arm studies, surrogate endpoints, or short-term outcomes. Last, because not every patient responds to the same treatment in the same way owing to heterogeneity of the patient population, it is of interest to both the patient and prescribing physician to understand potential effects of the treatment on an individual patient. In the traditional clinical trials, the efficacy and safety of a treatment is demonstrated through comparing the average outcomes of the treatment and control groups. Therefore, it does not provide the patient-specific assessments of efficacy and safety. That evidence generated from the traditional clinical research fails to guide patients, physicians, and health systems for real-world decisions, as noted by many researchers. Hand (2009) stressed that "the aim of a clinician is not really to work out whether drug A is superior to drug B 'on average,' but to enable a decision to be made about which drug to prescribe for the next patient who walks through the door, i.e., for the individual."

1.3 Real-World Data and Real-World Evidence

1.3.1 Real-World Data

RWD are data that are collected from diverse sources, outside the constraints of conventional RCT. They often consist of observational outcomes in a heterogeneous patient population. Because the data are not collected in a well-controlled experimental setting and come from diverse sources, they are likely unstructured, heterogeneous, complex, and inherently variable. RWD can be derived from electronic health records (EHRs), claims and billing activities, product and disease registries, patient-related activities in outpatient or in-home use settings, and health monitoring. They also may be captured through social media and wearable devices thanks to the advances of digital technologies. These latter data provide opportunities to deliver a holistic picture of an individual's health status and enable the patient to use one's own data for better adherence and disease management. RWD have the potential to drive a paradigm shift in healthcare from "drugs for disease" to "human engineering" where the care is personalized, based on patient and disease characteristics. Figure 1.2 displays various sources of RWD. The data source can be unstructured and noisy, and described in free text. As will be discussed later, the key to realizing the potential of RWD is to use quality data, valid statistical methods, and advanced analytics that can synthesize information from a large volume and diverse data sets.

1.3.2 Real-World Evidence

RWE is the clinical evidence regarding the usage and potential benefits or risks of a medical product derived from analysis of RWD from diverse sources

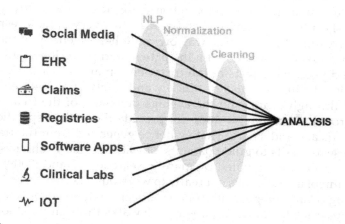

FIGURE 1.2
Sources of RWD. The Internet of Things (IOT) refers to physical devices that are connected to the Internet, collecting and sharing data.

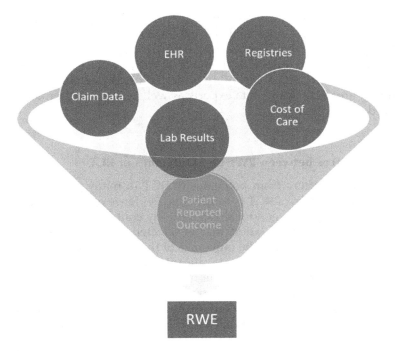

FIGURE 1.3
Generation of RWE from diverse sources of RWD.

as shown in Figure 1.3. RWE complements and enhances the evidence from RCTs, and provides information for decision-making throughout the product life cycle. The validity of RWE depends not only on the quality of RWD but also on the robustness of study design and appropriateness of statistical analysis.

Efforts have been made to blend the features of RCT with those of obervational studies. For example, pragmatic clinical trials (PCTs) utilize randomization in observational studies to produce quality RWE. Such studies have the potential to demonstrate the effectiveness of a drug at a greater reduced cost and time. Attempts have been made to provide guidance on how to run PCTs. For example, a tool kit for planning and conducting PCTs is provided on the PRECIS-2 website (PRECIS-2 2020). Control data derived from historical clinical trial data or RWD also can help mitigate confounding effects and minimize bias in the RWD, resulting in impoved quality of RWE. In addtion, RWE also can be dervied from hybrid designs, which combine design components of clinical effectiveness and implementation research (Curran et al. 2012). Zhu et al. (2020) discusses design considerations for hybrid trials and strategy to integrate hybrid trials in clinical programs.

The explosion of RWD and the need for insights, sometimes at the point of care, derived from these data entails the need to leverage advanced technologies to genereate RWE. Advances in technology such as natural language processing (NLP), artificial intelligence (AI), and machine learning (ML) provide such an opportunity. These tools allow extraction of data from unstructured sources with free-text. To fully capitalize on RWD, firms need to build robust RWE capability with dedicated personnel from interdiciplinary areas including data experts as well as analytical capability and enhanced data access.

1.3.3 Differences between RWE and Outcomes of RCT

Arguably, RWE differs from outcomes of RCT in many different aspects. The primary objective of RCT is to generate evidence of efficacy and safety of a new treatment. It is conducted in a highly controlled setting in a relatively homogeneous population that is selected based on a set of inclusion and exclusion criteria. The outcomes of the RCT are less variable, thus making it effective in detecting significant differences between the treatment and control. However, as previously discussed, the treatment effects such as efficacy do not necessarily translate into the effectiveness in the real-world setting as the subjects in the study may not be representative of the entire population. In contrast, the RWE can be used to show the effectiveness of the treatment in the diversified situations in the real-world setting. The differences between RCT and RWE are hightlighted in Table 1.1. In addition, RWE extracted from the RWD can be used to guide early drug discovery, clinical development, and healthcare decision-making by patients, prescibing physicians, and payers, which is disucssed in greater detail in Section 1.2.

TABLE 1.1

Differences between RCT and RWE

	RCT	RWE
Purpose	Efficacy/safety	Effectiveness/safety
Setting	Research	Real world
Population	Homogeneous	Heterogeneous
Population size	Small - moderate	Large - huge
Patient follow-up	Fixed	Variable
Treatment	Fixed	Variable
Attending physician	Investigator	Practitioner
Costs	High	Low
Generalizability	Low - moderate	Moderate - high
Control for bias	Design and conduct	Analysis

1.3.4 Regulatory Perspective

1.3.4.1 Productivity Challenge

In recent years, the biopharmaceutical industry has faced an unprecedented productivity challenge. Despite its high R&D spending that has soared to an unsustainable level, the number of new drug approvals has declined significantly. Many companies that rely on blockbuster drugs to generate revenue growth are in a bind due to patent expirations and the competition from generic drug and biosimilar makers. Meanwhile, consumers of biopharmaceutical products become more sophisticated and more demanding. Together, these challenges argue for disruptive innovations in both drug R&D and regulatory policies.

1.3.4.2 FDA Critical Path Initiative

On March 16, 2004, the FDA released a report, "Innovation/Stagnation: Challenge and Opportunity on the Critical Path to New Medical Products" (FDA 2004). From the FDA's viewpoint, the applied sciences needed for medical product development have not kept pace with the tremendous advances in the basic sciences. The new science is not being used to guide the technology development process in the same way that it is accelerating the technology discovery process. For medical technology, performance is measured in terms of product safety and effectiveness. Not enough applied scientific work has been done to create new tools to get fundamentally better answers about how the safety and effectiveness of new products can be demonstrated, in faster time frames, with more certainty, and at lower costs. In many cases, developers have no choice but to use the tools and concepts of the last century to assess this century's candidates. As a result, the vast majority of investigational products that enter clinical trials fail. Often, product development programs must be abandoned after extensive investment of time and resources. This high failure rate drives up costs, and developers are forced to use the profits from a decreasing number of successful products to subsidize a growing number of expensive failures. Finally, the path to market even for successful candidates is long, costly, and inefficient, due in large part to the current reliance on cumbersome assessment methods.

The report describes the urgent need to modernize the medical product development process—the Critical Path—to make product development more predictable and less costly. The report further points out that in an era of concerns about healthcare affordability, we need to make sure that new medical products are effective and provide accurate up-to-date information about using them so patients and doctors can make smart decisions about healthcare. As healthcare costs rise, patients, medical professionals, and healthcare purchasers are all demanding more value from the medical treatments they use. With more treatments in development than ever before, finding better ways to demonstrate their effectiveness for particular kinds of patients is essential for making sure that all Americans get the most value from their healthcare dollars.

Although use of RWD and RWE is not explicitly stated in the report as part of the new product development tool kit, it is apparent that companies not only need to improve the efficiency of target discovery and clinical trials but also influence patient, prescriber, and payer's options, as well as regulatory decisions, based on RWD, to ensure better patient outcome, accelerated approval, and greater market access.

1.3.4.3 Regulatory Perspectives Pertaining to RWE

1.3.4.3.1 U.S. Food and Drug Administration

The FDA considers RWD/RWE as a crucial component in regulatory reviews. Either through public announcements or publication of regulatory documents, the FDA has made the use of RWE as a key priority. In March 2016, the FDA released a statement regarding the objective and implementation of PDUFA. The statement indicated the use of RWE in regulatory decision-making.

In December 2016, the 21st Century Cures Act was signed into law (FDA 2016). The act is designed to help accelerate medical product development and bring new innovations and advances to patients who need them faster and more efficiently. It mandates the FDA to establish a program to evaluate the potential use of RWE to help support the approval of a new indication for an already approved drug or to help support or satisfy post-approval study requirements.

The FDA released a new strategic framework to advance the use of RWE to support development of drugs and biologics in December 2018 (FDA 2018c). The FDA's RWE program will evaluate the potential use of RWE to support changes to labeling about drug product effectiveness, including (1) adding or modifying an indication (e.g., change in dose, dose regimen, route of administration), (2) adding a new population, and (3) adding comparative effectiveness or safety information.

In the past several years, the FDA published several guidelines for the industry regarding use of RWE, including (1) "Submitting Documents Using Real-World Data and Real-World Evidence to the FDA for Drugs and Biologics Guidance for Industry" (FDA 2019b), (2) "Rare Diseases: Natural History Studies for Drug Development" (FDA 2019a), (3) "Use of Real-World Evidence to Support Regulatory Decision-Making for Medical Devices" (FDA 2017), and (4) "Final Guidance for Industry: Use of Electronic Health Record Data in Clinical Investigations" (FDA 2018a). In addition to the above guidelines that have already been issued, the FDA will be providing additional guidance documents including (1) guidance on how to assess whether RWD from medical claims, EHRs, and registries are fit for use to generate RWE to support effectiveness; (2) guidance for using RWD in RCTs for regulatory purposes, including pragmatic design elements; (3) guidance on the use of

RWD to generate external control arms; and (4) guidance about observation study designs, and how these might provide RWE to support effectiveness in regulatory decision-making.

Together, leveraging RWD/RWE for regulatory decisions is a key strategic priority for the FDA. While the FDA continues using RCT as the gold standard for generating evidence in support of regulatory decision-making, it is open to the use of RWD in clinical trials and willing to collaborate and explore the broader use of RWD in support of regulatory decision-making.

1.3.4.3.2 *European Medicines Agency (EMA)*

Historically, EMA has promoted use of RWD to complement and enhance evidence collected in RCTs especially for rare events and long-term outcomes (Higgins et al. 2013). In recent years, the agency also launched several initiatives to promote the use of high-quality RWD in decision-making. For example, in the document titled "EMA Regulatory Science to 2025 Strategic Reflection" published by the European Medicines Agency (EMA 2020), EMA has outlined a regulatory strategy for RWD. In addition, specific pilots of RWD analytics will be conducted, and work on pharmacovigilance methods will continue by (1) conducting a pilot of using rapid analytics of RWD (including EHRs) to support decision-making at the Pharmacovigilance Risk Assessment Committee (PRAC) and the Committee for Medicinal Products for Human Use (CHMP), (2) reviewing the utility of using EHRs for detecting drug safety issues (including drug interactions), and (3) mapping of good examples of RWD use in different phases of drug development to develop guidance on such use. Also of note is the regulatory approval tool called conditional approval, which is used in Europe, that grants marketing approval to enable early access of drugs targeting serious diseases for small patient populations or public emergencies (Martinalbo et al. 2016). Another tool used by the EMA for accelerating drug approval is Adaptive Pathways (EMA 2016a,b). It is founded on three principles: (1) iterative development, which either means approval in stages, beginning with a restricted patient population then expanding to wider patient populations, or confirming the benefit-risk balance of a product, following a conditional approval based on early data (using surrogate endpoints) considered predictive of important clinical outcomes; (2) gathering evidence through real-life use to supplement clinical trial data; and (3) early involvement of patients and health-technology–assessment bodies in discussions on a medicine's development.

Adaptive Pathways provides a framework for drug development and evidence generation in support of early patient access, taking advantage of existing tools including conditional approval.

Additionally, there were several presentations by scientific advisors of the EMA (Cave 2016; Royal College of General Practitioners 2018; Moseley 2018). However, although EMA recognized that considerable experience has been gained in using such data for pharmacovigilance, it also stressed that more experience is needed when using RWE to quantify the beneficial effects of medicines, either in reducing uncertainty post-approval, such as in Conditional Marketing Authorization, and for extending indications (Royal College of General Practitioners 2018). Hence, the role of RWE complementing pivotal RCT data for licensing dossiers remains uncertain. To progress, EMA needs RWE discussions on specific proposals. It also needs to encourage discussions among stakeholders including other decision makers and representatives (Moseley 2018).

On June 18–19, 2018, the EMA and FDA held their 2018 bilateral meeting in Brussels, Belgium, to review their ongoing cooperative initiatives, discuss strategic priorities for the coming years, and further strengthen the continuous close collaboration with specific action in the field of pharmaceuticals (EMA 2018). Among other topics, the use of RWE in regulatory decision-making was discussed. The EMA and FDA agreed that RWE holds major promise to strengthen decision-making on medicines throughout their life span. There are benefits from transatlantic collaboration to leverage expertise, experience, and available data. Collaboration will help to address methodological and practical challenges, and in analyzing RWE. The parties will collaborate on RWE, whereby EMA and FDA will regularly exchange information and work together on methodologies to optimize the use of RWE to support regulatory decision-making throughout the product life cycle. Thus far, the EMA has explored the use of RWD/RWE largely through several initiatives. They have not issued any guidelines. In general, their approach has been more conservative compared with those of the FDA.

1.3.4.3.3 *Health Canada (HC)*

In August 2018, HC initiated a project called Strengthening the Use of Real-World Evidence for Drugs that was aimed at improving the agency's ability to assess and monitor the safety, efficacy, and effectiveness of drugs across the drug life cycle (HC 2019a). HC intends to accomplish the objective by optimizing the use of RWE through stakeholder engagement. The taskforce of the project is responsible for (1) identifying opportunities for enhanced use of RWE throughout the drug life cycle, (2) mapping potential RWE sources, (3) developing and implementing an RWE strategy and implementation plan for the use of RWE in regulatory decision-making for drugs, and (4) consulting with stakeholders on the RWE strategy. The expected outcomes of the project include (1) increased use of RWE to enhance regulatory decision-making and risk communications throughout the drug life cycle, (2) improved use and sharing of RWE with healthcare system partners, (3) increased clarity for stakeholders on where and how RWE can be used to support regulatory decision-making, and (4) improved access to drugs through the use of new sources of evidence to support approval of drug applications.

On April 16, 2019, HC announced that they were working to optimize the use of RWE for regulatory decisions to improve the extent and rate of access to prescription drugs in Canada (HC 2019b). HC encourages RWE submissions (1) that aim to expand evidence-based indications for populations often excluded from clinical trials (e.g., children, seniors, and pregnant women); (2) for drugs/diseases in which clinical trials are unfeasible because they may be the case with rare diseases; and/or (3) in which clinical trials are unethical, as may be the case during emergencies in which dosages from animal studies may need to be extrapolated to treat humans potentially exposed to chemical or biological threats. At the same time, HC issued a guidance document titled "Elements of Real-world Data/Evidence Quality throughout the Prescription Drug Product Life Cycle" (HC 2019a). The aim of this document is to provide overarching principles to guide the generation of RWE that would be consistent with the regulatory standard of evidence in place in Canada and internationally. Although the agency noted that prospectively planned clinical trials have been and continue to be considered the most robust tool for providing evidence of drug safety and efficacy, they acknowledged that conducting clinical trials is not always feasible and thus may not always be deemed ethical for certain diseases/disorders (such as rare diseases) or patient populations, where excessive trial costs or small available patient populations may introduce constraints. Expanding data and evidence sources to include RWD/RWE may address some of these concerns and offer new opportunities to gain insight on public health, advance healthcare, and increase both the extent and rate of drug access for patient populations.

1.3.4.3.4 *Pharmaceuticals and Medical Devices Agency (PMDA)*

The perspective of Japan's PMDA on the use of RWD has been described by Uyama (2018). PMDA has utilized RWD for drug safety assessment since 2009. To promote greater use of RWD by pharmaceutical companies, PMDA amended it in October 2017 and implemented it on April 1, 2018. Accordingly, several related guidelines have been published recently, including (1) "Basic Principles on the Utilization of Health Information Databases for Post-Marketing Surveillance of Medical Products" (June 2017); (2) "General Steps for Considering a Plan of Post-Market Studies of a Drug" (January 2018); and (3) "Points to Consider for Ensuring Data Reliability on Post-Marketing Database Study for Drugs" (February 2018). In addition, the agency also launched MID-NET® (Medical Information Database Network) on April 1, 2018, which can be used by the pharmaceutical industry, academia, and the PMDA and its collaborative hospitals. The network is composed of 23 hospitals in 10 sentinel sites throughout Japan (Kondo 2017). Each sentinel site will establish a database of laboratory data, claim data, Diagnosis Procedure Combination (DPC) system data, and other data types, to be integrated by the PMDA into an analytical system that can extract and parse data in a tailored manner to meet specific purposes, and then compile and analyze the results. This was part of the "Rational Medicine" Initiative launched by the PMDA, aiming to create a patient-centric system, under which optimal medical care from the patient's point of view is provided.

Although the agency encourages the use of RWD, it also recognized several challenges, notably data quality, data coding, deep understanding about databases, validation of clinical outcomes and system infrastructure, timely and continuous communication with marketing authorization holders (MAH), and active collaborations among all stakeholders (Uyama 2018). It stresses the importance of experience and knowledge sharing among regulatory agencies and other stakeholders as the key step toward international harmonization in utilizing RWD in the regulatory process.

1.3.4.3.5 Other Countries

The important utility of RWE in support of accelerating cures and driving down overall healthcare costs is fully recognized by regulatory authorities in other regions. For example, in recent years, there has been increased use of RWE for healthcare decision-making (Sun 2019). The Indian government has also taken steps toward RWE by developing a framework to assist healthcare providers in harmonizing RWD for economic, clinical, and humanistic outcome (Dang and Vallish 2016).

1.3.4.4 Historical Approval Based on RWE

On April 4, 2019, the FDA approved Ibrance® (palbociclib) for the treatment of men with HR+, HER2- metastatic breast cancer, which was based predominately on RWD. The approval was based on data from EHRs and post-marketing reports of the real-world use of Ibrance® in male patients sourced from three real-world databases. This sets a precedence and paves the way for the future approvals of marketing applications. Thus far EMA has granted a handful of marketing authorization approvals, in which RWE was utilized to support regulatory decisions. Table 1.2 lists two examples.

It is worth noting that the historical approvals using RWE have largely been limited to (1) rare/orphan settings, (2) high unmet medical need, (3) RCTs not feasible or ethical, (4) no satisfactory treatment, (5) robust endpoint, and (6) substantial single-arm effect.

1.4 Access to RWD

RWD are collected from a large number of disparate sources, as discussed in Section 1.3. Three major types of RWD include EHRs, medical claims, and patient and disease registries. The development of EHRs has greatly enhanced the feasibility of collecting RWD and hamonizing the process, quality standards, and data management practice (Skovlund et al. 2018). A notable example is the InSite platform, the largest European live clinical data network, that enables trustworthy reuse of EHR data for research and efficient identification of patients who may be eligible for particular trials (InSite 2020). Recently, there have been sveral initiatives intended to develop new methods

TABLE 1.2

Examples of Market Authorization Approval by EMA Using Supportive RWE

Product and Indication	Pivotal Data	Driver for RWD Acceptability	Evidence Need	RWE Solutions
Axicabtagene ciloleucel (Yescarta) Adult patients with relapsed or refractory diffuse large B-cell lymphoma (DLBCL), primary mediastinal B-cell lymphoma (PMBCL) after two or more lines of systemic therapy.	Open-label, single-arm study (ZUMA 1 Phase II) with a primary endpoint of objective response rate defined as complete remission (CR) or partial remission (PR).[1]	• Rare disease • Orphan indication • Significant unmet need • RCT unfeasible	Need to provide confirmation of the pre-specified response rate of 20% and a historical context for interpreting the ZUMA 1 results. Additional evidence on long-term safety profile in post-marketing setting.	A retrospective patient-level pooled analysis of two Phase III RCTs and two observational studies (SCHOLAR 1) was developed as a companion study to contextualize the results of ZUMA 1. Further long-term follow-up of response and overall survival will be captured via a non-interventional post-authorization safety study (PASS) based on a registry.
Tisagenlecleucel (Kymriah) Adult patients with relapsed or refractory diffuse large B-cell lymphoma (DLBCL) after two or more lines of systemic therapy.	Open-label, single-arm study (C2201 Phase II) with a primary endpoint of overall response rate defined as the proportion of patients with CR or PR.[2]	• Rare disease • Orphan indication • Significant unmet need • RCT unfeasible	Need to provide confirmation of the pre-specified response rate of 20% and a historical context for interpreting the C2201 results. Additional evidence on long-term efficacy and safety.	Efficacy results compared against three external data sets (SCHOLAR 1, the CORAL extension study, PIX301) to contextualize the results of the single-arm trial. Further long-term follow-up of efficacy will be captured via a prospective observational study in patients with relapsed or refractory DLBCL based on data from a registry with efficacy outcomes similar to the C2201 study.

of RWE collection and synthesis for earlier adoption by the industry and health technology assessment (HTA) authorities. They include the Innovative Medicine Initiative's (IMI) GetReal (IMI 2020). Disease-based registries can be useful for understanding the natural history of diseases, assessing real-world safety, effectiveness, and cost-benefit (Garrison et al. 2007). Claim data, often collected retrospectively, are useful for cross-sectional analyses of clincal and economic outcomes, at patient, group, or population levels. They are great resources for phamracoeconomic assessments.

The majority of the RWD are privately owned while some are in the public domain. As discussed by Khosla et al. (2018), access to RWD falls into three categories, commericial, research collaboration, and developmental collaboration. The commerical data access is a fee-based option, acquired through a licensing agreement with heathcare informatics vendors. A firm can tap into the databases of the providers to address their research questions. Some large research organizations have their own database, which can be made accessible through research collaboration and agreement. Development data access focuses on developing one's own RWD through working with subject matter experts. Table 1.3 presents a list of RWD databases in various regions that house patient-level data in different therapeutic areas.

Table 1.4 lists key data fields in these databases.

In recent years, several initiatives have been launched to connect RWD from diverse sources and regions. Geldof et al. (2019) argued for the need of a

TABLE 1.3

Example Sources of RWD

Database	Type	Region	Therapeutic Areas
Truven MarketScan	Claim	US	All
CPRD	EMR	UK	All
Japan Medical Claim (JMDC/MDV)	Claim	Japan	Respiratory
NHANES (National Health and Nutrition Examination Survey)	Survey	US	All
Patient Like Me (PLM)	Patient-reported data	US	All
EHR4CR Insite Platform (Europe hospital network)	EMR	Pan-Europe	All
FlatIron	EMR	US	Oncology
CancerLinQ	EMR	US	Oncology
Symphony	Claim	US	Oncology
HealthVerity (HV)	EMR and claim	US	All
SEER	Registry	US	Oncology
Simulacrum	Registry	UK	Oncology
Diabetes Collaborative Registry (DCR)	Registry	US	Diabetes
Centricity	EMR	US	Diabetes
PINNACLE	Registry	US	Cardiovascular
Clipper	Registry and claim	US	Cardiovascular
Novelty (primary data collection)	Registry	Global	Respiratory
SPOCS (primary data collection)	Registry	Global	Lupus

TABLE 1.4

Key Data Fields in Medical Claim, EMS, and Registry

Key Data fields	Claim	EMR	Registry
Patient demographic	Yes	Yes	Yes
Vital signs	No	Yes	Yes
Diagnoses/conditions (ICD9/10)	Yes	Yes	Yes
Procedures	Yes	Yes	Yes
Lung function data	Few	Some	Yes
Lab test	Yes	Yes	Yes
Lab results	Few	Yes	Yes
Medications	Yes (pharmacy)	Yes (prescription)	Yes
Medications (details dosage, duration)	Some	Some	Yes
PRO	No	No	Yes
Provider notes (NLP)	No	Some	No
Biomarker	No	No	Yes
Symptom assessment	No	No ·	Yes
Mortality	Some	Some	Yes

federated RWD infrastructure to create a biomedical data ecosystem, which may satisfy the needs of (1) international data reusability, (2) real-time RWD processing, and (3) longitudinal RWD. To achieve these, a shift in data culture is needed, as are use cases demonstrating the value of multidisciplinary and cross-sector collaborations.

1.5 Opportunities of RWE in Drug Development

The confluence of RWD from disparate sources, such as genomic profiling, EHRs, medical claims, product and disease registries, patient-reported outcomes (PROs), health-monitoring devices, and so forth, together with AI and ML, has presented a plethora of opportunities to transform drug R&D to a more efficient and data-driven model, and to enable a new patient-centric development paradigm (Alemayehu and Berger 2016). Insights obtained from RWD/RWE can be used to aid key decision-making throughout the product life cycle (Khosla et al. 2018). Aided by data analytics, RWE has been transforming drug development and healthcare (Berger and Doban 2014; Alemayehu and Berger 2016; McDonald 2016; and Deloitte 2017). Some of the areas in which use of RWE is advantageous are shown in Figure 1.4.

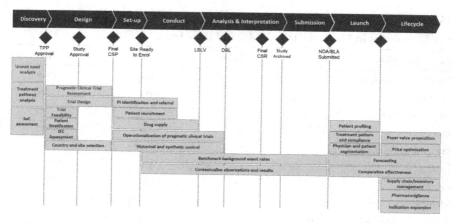

FIGURE 1.4

Use of RWE throughout the product life cycle. CSP, clinical study approval; CSR, clinical study report; DBL, database lock; IEC, independent ethics committee; LSLV, last subject last visit; NDA, new drug application; PI, principal investigator; SoC, standard of care; TPP, target product profile.

1.5.1 Early Discovery

In early discovery, RWE can be used to identify and profile patient populations for which there are unmet medical needs. In addition, through analysis of RWD, the treatment pathway for a target population can be mapped out, and effectiveness of the standard of care estimated. This information is helpful in informing decisions around the most appropriate drug development strategy, including determination of target product profile. RWE can be extremely useful in target discovery of oncology drug development, which has increasingly become personalized and precise. Combining genomic data with real-world clinical outcomes may create an opportunity to uncover biomarkers that can predict therapeutic response and disease resistance to the intervention, leading to a more targeted drug development strategy. Data collected from wearable devices, coupled with analytics, can provide real-time information about patient health status and enable the development of personalized medicine (Zheng et al. 2013).

1.5.2 Clinical Study Design and Feasibility

RWD have been historically and primarily used to help determine effect and sample sizes for powering RCTs. Use of RWE can help assess the impact of inclusion and exclusion criteria on trial feasibility and inform selection of site/country. Moreover, RWE also can be used to determine prognostic indications or baseline characteristics for patient stratification. For innovative trial designs that utilize Bayesian methods, RWE can be used to construct informative priors for the control, resulting in greater efficiency in study design and data analysis. Predictive markers derived from real-world sources can enable enrichment trial design and can potentially be used as surrogate endpoints.

Many of the concerns about the use of RWE are centered on the quality of RWD and validity of the findings. PCTs, conducted using less constrained study designs and broader populations, can serve as a bridge between evidence from RWD sources and RCTs. PCTs utilize the fundamental principles of patient randomization in a controlled trial setting with pre-specified follow-up, using more inclusive and representative population than a typical RCT. PCTs do not require strict adherence to study protocol to mimic the use of the product in the real-world. When properly designed, they can generate evidence to inform both regulatory and payer decision-making. Several PCTs have been successfully conducted, including the Salford Lung Studies (SLS) (Vestbo et al. 2016; Woodcock et al. 2017). The outcomes of the SLS studies were accepted by the EMA and deemed to have fulfilled the post-approval commitment.

RWD can be leveraged to support country selection for a trial targeting a rare disease. For example, one top pharmaceutical company designed a trial to quantify the impact of one of its oncology drugs on non-small cell lung cancer (NSCLC) patients with a comorbidity. Because the condition is rare, underdiagnosed, and prognosis is poor on diagnosis, it presents a very challenging environment for patient recruitment. Using networks on EHR in different regions, the company evaluated the best countries in which to conduct the trial based on (1) the eligible patient population, (2) ease of recruitment, and (3) saturation with other trials targeting a similar patient population. The effort led to the selection of countries in which they were able to recruit patients most efficiently.

1.5.3 Study Execution

RWE has the potential to improve planning and execution of clinical trials, including data-driven design to decrease clinical trial protocol amendments, accelerated patient recruitment through identifying patients, using analytics and selecting fast enrolling sites based on past performance such as the number of violations, and risk-based monitoring to mitigate data quality issues. RWD can be leveraged to predict the demand for drug supply of ongoing trials. Adequate drug supply is important for the successful completion of the trials. On the other hand, drugs have a certain shelf-life, so overproduction is very costly. Given that drug manufacturing usually takes 9–12 months, it is crucial to estimate the demand at least a year in advance. Using Bayesian analysis, which combines the historical data from similar trials with the patient retention in the current data, may provide accurate estimations of drug supply required to complete the trial.

For rare diseases and many oncology trials, it is often operationally unfeasible and unethical to conduct RCTs. There are growing needs to generate supportive evidence for the safety and effectiveness of a new drug from other sources such as observational studies. A synthetic control arm derived from historical or contemporaneous populations treated in a real-world setting may serve as a comparator for the experimental drug. Much research has been conducted to establish a valid external control (see Chapter 4). The commonly used strategies for inferring causal relationship from observational data are reviewed in Chapter 7.

1.5.4 Marketing Application

RWE was traditionally used in the regulatory process through pharmacovigilance programs to understand the safety of a drug in the context of its use in the real world rather than the controlled setting of RCTs. As previously discussed in Section 1.3, there is increasing interest in the use of RWE to support regulatory decision-making (Cave et al. 2019). RWD were used for detecting long-term safety concerns as well as disease characterization and prevalence, understanding current standard of care, and confirming the clinical outcome of short-term surrogate markers (Cave et al. 2019). As more drugs are approved by regulatory authorities either through the FDA orphan drug and breakthrough therapy designations (FDA 2004) or EMA Conditional Approval (Martinalbo et al. 2016) or Adaptive Pathways (EMA 2016a,b), using RWE to supplement the findings in RCTs helps avoid costly post-marketing trials and ensures early access. A prime example is the FDA's recent approval of Tagrisso™ for NSCLC patients with EFGR T790M mutation, on the condition that the sponsor would provide overall response data from real-world patients given the treatment (FDA 2018b). As noted by Chatterjee et al. (2018), this conditional approval of Tagrisso™ by the FDA may represent an emerging regulatory mechanism, which encourages the use of post-marketing requirements to fill evidence gaps from RCTs. Several other examples of early approval are presented in Eichler et al. (2008), Banzi et al. (2015), Lipska et al. (2015), and Hoekman et al. (2016).

1.5.5 Product Launch

Although RCTs remain the gold standard for gaining regulatory approval, getting regulatory approval of a new drug is not enough as there are many questions that are not addressed by the data from RCTs. For example, it is uncertain how the drug may work in populations or under conditions not studied in the RCTs or relative to other drugs in targeting the same populations not yet evaluated in the studies (Garrison et al. 2007). To capture return on investment (ROI), the drugs must generate revenue. To do that, prescribers must be willing to prescribe the drug (over competitors' drugs), payers must be willing to reimburse it, and patients must be willing to stay on it (and not drop out and switch to another drug after a short time). Thus, the evidence has to show that a large proportion of patients benefit from the drug (and they do so better than on a competitor's drug). Comparative effectiveness of the drug based on RWE that goes beyond information collected from RCTs has been increasingly utilized by healthcare decision-makers for making treatment, coverage, and payment decisions and helping physicians/patients make informed decisions at the point of care. In addition, companies also seek RWE outcomes to understand treatment patterns and adherence, gain information on competitors, and target underserved patient groups.

RWE also plays a key role in forecasting the demands for drugs, increasing operation efficiency and reducing costs. To gain competitive advantages, a pharmaceutical company needs to understand the characteristics of patients who are given their drugs, treatment pattern and compliance, and profiles of physicians so that they can conduct targeted branding and marketing. One pharmaceutical company developed a mobile application for the sales force of their respiratory drug. Using a predictive algorithm and patient blood tests at the point of care, the mobile application predicts in real time if the patient is suitable for the drug. This allows the sales representative to recommend the use of the product directly to the attending physician.

1.5.6 Product Life Cycle Management

From the product life cycle management perspective, effective insights gleaned from RWD bring about payer value propositions. Various methods for value assessments have been proposed by stakeholders such as payers and HTA agencies (see Chapter 6 for a detailed discussion). Evidence from observational studies can fill in the efficacy-effective gap as previously discussed. Demands for the new drugs and a better understanding of competitors' products based on RWD can help optimize drug price and bring about efficiency of the drug supply, drug supply chain, and inventory management. For example, the analysis of RWD can lead to a better understanding of key performance indices of the supply chain such as delayed shipment and help to identify key areas for improvement.

Pharmacovigilance is also an important aspect of product life cycle management. Increasingly, greater attention has been given to data from secondary sources for the detection of a safety signal of rare events (Finkel et al. 2014; Alemayehu and Berger 2016). In May 2008, the FDA launched the Sentinel Initiative, which is a long-term program designed to build and implement RWD network for monitoring the safety of FDA-approved drugs and other medical products (FDA 2010). The systems include data from a wide range of sources including EHR and claims data. In certain instances, the use of RWD for pharmacovigilance was shown to be advantageous in revealing hidden safety signals compared with the traditional methods (Gooden et al. 2013).

Last, RWE can be used to aid in risk and benefit assessment of populations that are historically not included in RCTs. There have been several successful regulatory approvals for label expansion, based on RWE, including the FDA approval of Ibrance® (palbociclib) for the treatment of men with HR+, HER2 metastatic breast cancer.

1.6 Challenges with RWE

With the successes of RWE used in various aspects of drug product life cycle, there is tremendous enthusiasm and growing hope to transform the way new medicines are developed. However, use of RWE also raises a multitude of unique challenges. If not properly addressed, these challenges may compromise the validity of conclusions drawn from the RWE on product safety and efficacy.

1.6.1 Data Access and Quality

The legal and ethical requirements for sharing data vary from region to region. At present, there is no clear regulatory and legal framework for sharing data from multinational sources. The reluctance of pharmaceutical companies and healthcare organizations to share their clinical data creates additional data gaps. All of these hamper the implementation of RWE strategy.

Another issue regarding RWD is around data quality. RWD are collected in a routine healthcare setting and from various sources. Unlike data from RCTs, RWD are not routinely monitored and curated according to pre-specified quality standards to ensure correctness, accuracy, and completeness. Data may suffer from omissions or misclassification. Numerous other data issues exist, including varying terminology and perception of quality in different regions. In addition, bias may be introduced due to a variety of reasons such as miscoding of treatment (Hampson et al. 2018), misclassification of the cause of death (Skovlund et al. 2018), and reporting of bias (McGauran et al. 2010).

To realize the full value of RWD, the data must meet certain quality standards. RWD are usually curated retrospectively before their use. However, such an effort can be both time consuming and costly. It also may introduce errors and biases. The lack of existing regulatory guidance on the RWD quality issues only exacerbates the situation. The problem is fully recognized by the regulatory agency. Currently, the FDA is developing guidelines on data quality issues unique to the RWD setting and related study design considerations (Brennan 2019).

1.6.2 Technological Barriers

As noted by various researchers (Alemayehu and Berger 2016; Cave 2016; Skovlund et al. 2018), the heterogeneity comes from the large volume, unstructured nature, and sometimes real-time collection of RWD entailing new technological platforms and solutions for access, analysis, integration, and visualization of complex data sets. A technological build may require a significant amount of investment and can be a daunting task. Another issue is validation of various devices such as wearable devices that collect real-time data of an individual patient's health status (Alemayehu and Berger 2016). There is no coherent effort to validate these devices.

1.6.3 Methodological Challenges

In RCTs, randomization ensures both variables measured or not measured in the studies are balanced across study group. It mitigates the potential cofounding effect caused by the variables that underscore the validity of statistical tests used to compare treatments. However, confounding is inherent in data from nonrandomized studies regardless of data quality, and interpreting treatment effect becomes challenging if not at all impossible.

As discussed by Skovlund et al. (2018), there are several remedies that can be used to control for potential confounding. One is to adjust for known confounding factors through statistical models. However, there exist so-called residual confounding caused by factors that are not measured or measurement error due to misclassification of the known confounding variables (Greenland 1996; Skovlund et al. 2018). Another potential solution is to use propensity score-based methods to match patients to different treatments according to key patient characteristics (see Chapters 4 and 7 for detailed discussion). But propensity scores also suffer the inability to balance characteristics that are not measured (Rubin 1997). The use of instrumental variables as a substitute for the actual treatment status is another alternative method, but it has its own challenges. For instance, it is difficult to find such valid instruments (Greenland 2000; Schneeweiss 2007; Burgess and Thompson 2011).

As discussed by Hampson et al. (2018), various efforts have been made to establish best practices and standards for collecting and analyzing RWE (Greenfield and Kaplan 2012; Montori et al. 2012; Garrison et al. 2007; NCP 2017). However, there is still lack of agreement in the published literature on best practices for the generation of RWE.

1.6.4 Lack of Data Talents

Data scientists are a new breed of analytical experts in extracting insights from complex data sets to aid business decision-making. To be effective, data scientists have to have solid grounding in statistics, computer sciences including AI, and ML, as well as domain knowledge in various aspects of drug development. Currently, there is clear lack of data science expertise in pharmaceutical and healthcare industries. Few academic institutions provide data science programs. RWD are often analyzed by inexperienced personnel. This may cause concerns in the robustness of methods used and validation of the RWE drawn from such data.

1.6.5 Regulatory Risks

Despite the advances in regulatory policy and successful case examples of regulatory approvals for label expansion and new indications based on RWE, there is no clear regulatory pathway regarding marketing approval based on RWE. This is in part due to the continued prevailing regulatory view that RCT remains the gold standard for generating evidence to support licensure applications. The concerns of data quality, and methodological and technological barriers impose additional challenges in adopting RWD in regulatory decision-making. There is a need to address these issues to enhance the robustness and quality of RWE generated.

1.7 Concluding Remarks

In the last decade, the pharmaceutical industry has faced an unprecedented productivity challenge. Despite many innovations in biomedical research that created a plethora of opportunities for detection, treatment, and prevention of serious illnesses, a high percentage of candidate drugs showing promise in early research have failed in late stages of clinical development. Meanwhile, there have been growing demands for pharmaceutical companies to demonstrate value to payers and health authorities. Successful drug development relies on not only the sponsor's ability to leverage advances in science and technology, but also the ability to use RWE to gain marketing approval, optimize pricing, and influence coverage decisions. The recent development of governmental policies and guidelines has brought about more clarity on the use of RWE to aid drug development and healthcare decision-making. Aided by digital technologies, advanced analytics, and more collaborative and open regulatory environments, RWE has made many successful strides throughout drug product life cycles and will continue to be at the forefront of medical innovations. However, there still remain numerous methodological, technical, ethical, and regulatory challenges. The resolutions of these issues require effort from multiple stakeholders. To capitalize on RWE and thrive in a value-focused environment of changing technology and evolving regulations, firms need to embrace a new drug development paradigm based on a holistic way of evidence generation from target discovery, through clinical development and regulatory approval to commercialization. This includes establishing an effective data governance strategy with well-defined structure and processes to ensure robust data infrastructure; leveraging technology platforms for access, analysis, integration and visualization of heterogeneous data sets; and using advanced analytics based on AI and ML to translate RWD into actionable insights.

References

Alemayehu, D. and Berger, M.L. 2016. Big Data: transforming drug development and health policy decision making. *Health Services & Outcomes Research Methodology*, 16, 92–102.

Banzi, R., Gerardi, C., Bertele, V., Garattini, S. 2015. Approvals of drugs with uncertain benefit-risk profiles in Europe. *Eur. J. Intern. Med.* 26, 572–584. 10.1016/j.ejim.2015.08.008

Barton, S. 2000. Which clinical studies provide the best evidence?: the best RCT still trumps the best observational. *BMJ*, 321(7256), 255–256.

Berger, M.L. and V. Doban. 2014. Big data, advanced analytics and the future of comparative effectiveness research study. *Journal of Comparative Effectiveness Research*, 3(2), 167–176.

Black, N. 1996. Why we need observational studies to evaluate effectiveness of health care. *BMJ*, 312, 1215–1218.

Brennan, Z. 2019. FDA developing guidance on real-world data quality issues, officials say. https://www.raps.org/news-and-articles/news-articles/2019/9/fda-developing-guidance-on-real-world-data-quality.

Burgess, S. and Thompson, S.G. 2011. Avoiding bias from weak instruments in Mendelian randomization studies. *International Journal of Epidemiology*, 40, 755–764.

Cave, A. 2016. What are the real-world evidence tools and how can they support decision making? EMA-EuropaBio Info Day, November 22, 2016. https://www.ema.europa.eu/en/documents/presentation/presentation-what-are-real-world-evidence-tools-how-can-they-support-decision-making-dr-alison-cave_en.pdf. Accessed June 7, 2019.

Cave, A., Kurz, X., and Arlett, P. 2019. Real-world data for regulatory decision making: challenges and possible solutions for Europe. *Clinical Pharmacology & Therapeutics*, 106(1), 36–39. DOI:10.1002/cpt.1426.

Chatterjee, A., Chilukuri, S., Fleming, E., Knepp, A., Rathore, S., and Zabinski, J. 2018. Real-world evidence: driving a new drug development paradigm in oncology. https://www.mckinsey.com/industries/pharmaceuticals-and-medical-products/our-insights/real-world-evidence-driving-a-new-drug-development-paradigm-in-oncology. Accessed June 11, 2019.

Curran, G.M., Bauer, M., Mittman, B., Pyne, J.M., and Stetler, C. 2012. Effectiveness-implementation hybrid designs - combining elements of clinical effectiveness and implementation research to enhance public health impact. *Medical Care*, 50(3), 217–226.

Dang, A. and Vallish, B.N. 2016. Real-world evidence: an Indian perspective. *Perspectives in Clinical Research*, 7(4), 156–160.

Deloitte. 2017. Getting real with real-world evidence Deloitte's Real-World Evidence Benchmark Survey shows life sciences companies have room for improvement. https://www2.deloitte.com/content/dam/Deloitte/us/Documents/life-sciences-health-care/us-ls-2017-real-world-evidence-survey-031617.pdf. Accessed June 12, 2019.

EMA. 2016a. Final report on the adaptive pathways pilot. https://www.ema.europa.eu/en/documents/report/final-report-adaptive-pathways-pilot_en.pdf. Accessed June 13, 2019.

EMA. 2016b. Guidance for companies considering the adaptive pathways approach. Guidance for companies considering the adaptive pathways approach. https://www.ema.europa.eu/en/documents/regulatory-procedural-guideline/guidance-companies-considering-adaptive-pathways-approach_en.pdf. Accessed June 11, 2019.

EMA. 2018. Reinforced EU/US collaboration on medicines. https://www.ema.europa.eu/en/news/reinforced-euus-collaboration-medicines. Accessed June 7, 2019.

EMA. 2020. EMA Regulatory Science to 2025: Strategic reflection. https://www.ema.europa.eu/en/documents/regulatory-procedural-guideline/ema-regulatory-science-2025-strategic-reflection_en.pdf. Accessed June 10, 2020.

Eichler, H.G., Pignatti, F., Flamion, B., et al. (2008). Balancing early market access to new drugs with the need for benefit/risk data: a mounting dilemma. *Nat Rev Drug Discov*, 7, 818–826.

FDA. 2004. Innovation/Stagnation: Challenge and Opportunity on the Critical Path to New Medical Products. https://c-path.org/wp-content/uploads/2013/08/FDACPIReport.pdf. Accessed June 7, 2019.

FDA. 2010. The Sentinel Initiative. https://www.fda.gov/media/79652/download. Accessed June 11, 2019.

FDA. 2016. 21st Century Cures Act. https://www.fda.gov/regulatory-information/selected-amendments-fdc-act/21st-century-cures-act. Accessed June 7, 2019.

FDA. 2017. Use of Real-World Evidence to Support Regulatory Decision-Making for Medical Devices. https://www.fda.gov/regulatory-information/search-fda-guidance-documents/use-real-world-evidence-support-regulatory-decision-making-medical-devices. June 7, 2019.

FDA. 2018a. Final Guidance for Industry: Use of Electronic Health Record Data in Clinical Investigations. https://www.fda.gov/drugs/news-events-human-drugs/final-guidance-industry-use-electronic-health-record-data-clinical-investigations-12062018-12062018. Accessed June 11, 2019.

FDA. 2018b. Postmarket requirements and commitments. http://www.accessdata.fda.gov/scripts/cder/pmc/index.cfm. June 11, 2019.

FDA. 2018c. Statement from FDA Commissioner Scott Gottlieb, M.D., on FDA's new strategic framework to advance use of real-world evidence to support development of drugs and biologics. https://www.fda.gov/news-events/press-announcements/statement-fda-commissioner-scott-gottlieb-md-fdas-new-strategic-framework-advance-use-real-world. Accessed June 7, 2019.

FDA. 2019a. Rare Diseases: Natural History Studies for Drug Development. https://www.fda.gov/media/122425/download. January 7, 2020.

FDA. 2019b. Submitting Documents Using Real-World Data and Real-World Evidence to FDA for Drugs and Biologics Guidance for Industry. https://www.fda.gov/media/124795/download. January 7, 2020.

Finkle, W.D., Greenland, S., Ridgeway, G.K., Adams, J.L., Frasco, M.A., Cook, M.B., et al. 2014. Increased risk of non-fatal myocardial infarction following testosterone therapy prescription in men. *PLoS One*, 9(1), e85805. doi:10.1371/journal.pone.0085805

Garrison Jr, L.P., Neumann, P.J., Erickson, J., Marshall, D., and Mullins, D. 2007. Using real-world data for coverage and payment decisions: The ISPOR Real-World DataTask Force Report. *Value in Health*, 10(5), 326–335.

Geldofl, T., Huys, I, and Dyck, W.V. 2019. Real-world evidence gathering in oncology: the need for a biomedical big data insight-providing federated network. Front. Med., https://doi.org/10.3389/fmed.2019.00043. Accessed January 7 2020.

Gooden, K.M., Pan, X., Kawabata, H., et al. 2013. Use of an algorithm for identifying hidden drug–drug interactions in adverse event reports. *Journal of the American Medical Informatics Association*, 20, 590.

Greenfield, S. and Kaplan, S.H. 2012. Building useful evidence: changing the clinical research paradigm to account for comparative effectiveness research. *Journal of Comparative Research*, 1(3), 263–270. DOI: https://doi.org/10.2217/cer.12.23.

Greenland, S. 1996. Basic methods for sensitivity analysis of biases. *International Journal of Epidemiology*, 25, 1107–1116.

Greenland, S. 2000. An introduction to instrumental variables for epidemiologists. *International Journal of Epidemiology*, 29, 722–729.

Hampson, G., Towse, A., Dreitlein, W.B., Henshall, C., and Pearson, S.D. 2018. Real-world evidence for coverage decisions: opportunities and challenges. *Journal of Comparative Effectiveness Research*, 7(12), 1133–1143.

HC. 2019a. Elements of Real-world Data/Evidence Quality throughout the Prescription Drug Product Life Cycle. https://www.canada.ca/en/services/health/publications/drugs-health-products/real-world-data-evidence-drug-lifecycle-report.html. Accessed January 7, 2020.

HC. 2019b. Optimizing the Use of Real-world Evidence to Inform Regulatory Decision-Making. https://www.canada.ca/en/health-canada/services/drugs-health-products/drug-products/announcements/optimizing-real-world-evidence-regulatory-decisions.html. Accessed January 7, 2020.

Higgins, J.P., Ramsay, C., Reeves, B.C., et al. 2013. Issues relating to study design and risk of bias when including non-randomized studies in systematic reviews on the effect of interventions. *Research Synthesis Methods*, 3(4), 603–612.

Hoekman J., Klamer T.T., Mantel-Teeuwisse, A.K., et al. Characteristics and follow-up of postmarketing studies of conditionally authorized medicines in the EU. *Br J Clin Pharmacol*, 82, 213–226.

IMI. 2020. Europe's Partnership for Health. https://www.imi.europa.eu/. Accessed January 7, 2020.

InSite. 2020. The Largest European Live Clinical Data Network. https://www.insiteplatform.com/. Accessed January 7, 2020.

Khosla, S., White, R., Medina, J., Ouwens, M., Emmas, C., Koder, T., Male, G., and Lenoard, S. 2018. Real-world evidence (RWE) – a disruptive innovation or the quiet evolution of medical evidence generation. *F1000Research*, 7, 1–13.

Kondo, T. 2017. "Rational Medicine" Initiative. https://www.pmda.go.jp/files/000216304.pdf. Accessed June 7, 2019.

Lipska, I. Hoekman, J., McAuslane, N., Leufkens, H.G.M., Hövels, A. M., 2015. Does conditional approval for new oncology drugs in Europe lead to differences in health technology assessment decisions? *Clinical Pharmacology & Therapeutics*, 98(5), 489–491.

Martinalbo, J. Bowen, D., and Camarero, J. and et al. 2016. Early market access of cancer drugs in the EU. *Annals of Oncology*, 27(1), 96–105.

McDonald, L., Lambrelli, D., Wasiak, R. and Ramagopalan, S.V. 2016. Real-world data in the United Kingdom: opportunities and challenges. BMC Medicine,14. https://bmcmedicine.biomedcentral.com/articles/10.1186/s12916-016-0647-x. Accessed January 7 2020.

McGauran, N., Beate, W., Kreis, J., Schuler, Y.B., Kolsch, H., and Kaiser, T. 2010. Reporting bias in medical research – a narrative review. *Trials*, 11(37). DOI: 10.1186/1745-6215-11-37.

Montori, V.M., Kim, S.P., Guyatt, G.H., and Shah, N.D. 2012. Which design for which question? An exploration toward a translation table for comparative effectiveness research. *Journal of Comparative Effectiveness Research*, 1(3), 271–279. DOI: https://doi.org/10.2217/cer.12.24.

Moseley J. 2018. Regulatory Perspective on Real-world Evidence (RWE) in Scientific Advice. https://www.ema.europa.eu/en/documents/presentation/presentation-regulatory-perspective-real-world-evidence-rwe-scientific-advice-emas-pcwp-hcpwp-joint_en.pdf. June 7, 2019.

NPC. 2017. Standards for Real-World Evidence. http://www.npcnow.org/issues/evidence/standards-for-real-world-evidence. Accessed June 11, 2019.

PRECIS-2. 2020. The PRECIS-2 Website has Two Functions. http://www.precis-2.org/. Accessed June 12, 2020.

Royal College of General Practitioners. 2018. BIA/MHAR Conference Report. https://www.bioindustry.org/uploads/assets/uploaded/2ceb87ee-bd78-4549-94bff0655fffa5b6.pdf. Accessed June 7, 2019.

Rubin, D.B. 1997. Estimating causal effects from large data sets using propensity scores. *Annals of Internal Medicine*, 127, 757–763.

Schneeweiss, S. 2007. Development in post-marketing comparative effectiveness research. *Clinical Pharmacology and Therapeutics*, 82, 143–156.

Skovlund et al. (2018). The use of real-world data in cancer drug development. *European Journal of Cancer*, 1010, 69–76.

Sun, X. 2019. Real-world evidence in China - Current practices, challenges, strategies and developments. https://www.ispor.org/docs/default-source/conference-ap-2018/china-2nd-plenary-for-handouts.pdf. Accessed June 12, 2019.

Uyama, Y. 2018. Utilizing Real-World Data: A PMDA Perspective. Proceedings of DIA 2019 Annual Meeting. https://globalforum.diaglobal.org/issue/august-2018/utilizing-real-world-data-a-pmda-perspective/. Accessed June 7, 2019.

Vestbo, J., Leather, D., Bakerly, N., et al. 2016. Effectiveness of fluticasone furoate – vilanterol for COPD in clinical practice. *NEJM*, 357, 1253–1260.

Woodcock, A., Vestbo, J., Bakerly N., et al. 2017. Effectiveness of fluticasone furoate plus vilanterol on asthma control in clinical practice: an open-label, parallel group, randomised controlled trial. *Lancet*, 390(10109), 2247–2255.

Zheng, J., Shen, Y., Zhang, Z., Wu, T., Zhang, G., and Lu, H. 2013. Emerging wearable medical devices towards personalized healthcare. In Proceedings of the 8th International Conference on Body Area Networks. https://eudl.eu/doi/10.4108/icst.bodynets.2013.253725. Accessed June 11, 2019.

Zhu, M., Sridhar, S., Hollingworth, R., Chit, A., Kimball, T., Murmell, K., Greenberg, M, Gurunathan, S., Chen, J. 2020. Hybrid clinical trials to generate real-world evidence: design considerations from a sponsor's perspective. *Contemporary Clinical Trials*, 94, 105856. DOI: 10.1016/j.cct.2019.105856

2

Evidence Derived from Real-World Data: Utility, Constraints, and Cautions

Deepak B. Khatry

There is growing interest in greater utilization of evidence generated from data sources other than randomized controlled trials (RCTs) to inform treatment decisions on patients and to improve overall healthcare. These data, which originate from non-RCT sources such as routine clinical practice, patient registries, and observational studies, are referred to as "real-world data (RWD)." Evidence synthesized from such RWD is referred to as "real-world evidence (RWE)." An implicit assumption for reliability and validity of RWE will be an adequate assurance of quality of both the RWD and the RWE. Benefits from the use of RWE could accrue

1. directly to patients such as through new evidence of efficacy and/or safety of therapies or by more appropriate pairing of patients with available treatments (i.e., improvements in precision medicine) and
2. indirectly from using such evidence for more efficient designs of clinical trials that lead to higher probabilities of success, more efficient regulatory approvals of new drugs for earlier patient access, improvements in coverage reimbursement approvals from payers, and increased efficiency in use of overall societal healthcare resources.

Quality evaluations and assurances must be made on two fronts: (1) RWD, which represents measured patient attributes, and (2) RWE, which must be derived by meeting standards of appropriateness of study designs and statistical methods and tests used to synthesize and summarize applicable findings from the RWD. As RWE is derived from RWD, we must first ensure the quality and validity of RWD. In this chapter, I discuss opportunity and constraints related to RWD and RWE from my review of the latest scientific literature together with the incorporation of my perspectives on the topic that is additionally informed by my own research. I will conclude by summarizing cautions and recommendations related to standards of quality assurances in RWD and the evidence generated from such data.

When properly designed and implemented, sample surveys have external validity, and results obtained from such studies can be generalized to the representative populations of interest. Carefully designed studies such as well-controlled laboratory experiments, in contrast, have internal validity, and results from such studies support causal inferences to be made. Ideally, combining both types of research, which has been termed in social sciences and psychological research as "survey experiments," has the potential to generate results that will have both internal and external validity, and possess potential to infer causal relationships that may be generalizable. A good reference on the design and application of survey experiments in the social sciences is the book by Mutz (2011). Mutz challenges conventional wisdom about internal and external validity of studies and demonstrates that strong causal claims need not come at the expense of external validity, and that it will be possible to execute experiments remotely using large population samples. In theory, RWD could be used for such purposes in biomedicine.

In the development and use of medicines, pragmatic trials have been proposed as one way to design studies to generate generalizable evidence while maintaining methodological purity by balancing internal and external validity (Godwin et al. 2003). Two decades ago, Roland and Torgerson published a clinical review in the *British Medical Journal* in which they made a distinction between what they termed as "explanatory" trials (such as RCTs), which measure "efficacy" of a new treatment, and "pragmatic" trials, which measure "effectiveness," defined as "benefit the treatment produces in routine clinical trials" (Roland and Torgerson 1998). The topic of pragmatic trials is currently of considerable interest. In a recent review article in the *New England Journal of Medicine*, Ford and Norrie (2016) referenced a special issue of the journal *Clinical Trials*, which contained 12 articles focusing on ethical and regulatory issues in pragmatic trials. Another series of eight articles entitled *"Pragmatic Trials and Real World Evidence"* has been published by the *Journal of Clinical Epidemiology*. In the first of those eight papers, Zuidgeest et al. (2017a) integrated the theoretical design options with the practice of conducting pragmatic trials. In the second paper, Worsley et al. (2017) described the challenges in the selection of sites for pragmatic trials and the impact on validity, precision, and generalizability of the results. In the third paper, Rengerink et al. (2017) addressed the challenges of identifying, enrolling, and retaining participants in trials conducted within routine clinical care settings. In the fourth paper, Kalkman et al. (2017) explored pragmatic trials as one way to generate evidence in routine care settings that align with aims of the GetReal consortium of the Innovative Medicines Initiative aimed at developing strategies to incorporate RWE earlier into the drug life cycle. The fifth paper by Zuidgeest et al. (2017b) discusses the usual care as a comparator and allocation of treatment strategies. In the sixth paper, Welsing et al. (2017) discussed different types of outcomes and their suitability for pragmatic trials, design choices for measuring such outcomes, and their implications and challenges. In the seventh paper, Irving et al. (2017) focused on the impact of design choices on the practical implementation of pragmatic trials. In the final and eighth paper, Meinecke et al. (2017) focused on challenges and solutions for data collection and management in pragmatic trials in which a high level of accuracy and completeness of data need to be balanced with a low level of interference with clinical practice. This series of eight articles is an excellent resource for researchers and practitioners who are interested in understanding and planning real-world studies (RWSs) with aims to generate RWE.

Ford and Norrie (2016) provided a more general perspective on the promise and limitations of pragmatic trials:

> No single trial, pragmatic or otherwise, is likely to answer all potential questions about the value of any healthcare technology. A pragmatic approach to pragmatism would be to adopt the features of pragmatic trials whenever feasible and sensible, and when such features do not compromise trial quality and the ability to answer the clinical question of interest.

Thus, the hurdle for satisfying both internal and external validities when using RWD and generating RWE are quite high. To investigate how well observational data can be used to address the same clinical questions answered by traditional clinical trials, Bartlett et al. (2019) studied clinical trials published in 2017 in high-impact journals that could be feasibly replicated using observational data from insurance claims and/or electronic health records (EHRs). They found that only 15% (33/220) of the trials in their study could be feasibly replicated through administrative claims or EHR data. Thus, although there is potential for RWE to complement clinical trials, the authors caution that using observational methods and data sources is not feasible for examining safety and efficacy of a medical product that is not in widespread use in routine clinical practice. My own perspective is that, in the present, RWD and RWE can mostly be used to supplement evidence of drug efficacy accrued from RCTs and to investigate generalizability to the real-world population. This may change in the future if improvements can be made in quality and capture of RWD. The rest of this chapter is organized into the following six sections for additional discussion: (1) What is RWD in the Context of Drug Development and Clinical Practice?, (2) Why Is RWD Important?, (3) For What Purposes Can RWD Be Useful?, (4) What Study Designs and Statistical Methods Will Be Necessary to Ensure High-Quality RWE?, (5) Some Application Examples, and (6) Summary.

2.1 What Is RWD in the Context of Drug Development and Clinical Practice?

RWD and RWE are increasingly recognized as important terms in the synthesis of clinically relevant information to advance healthcare. The landscape associated with these two terms in the scientific literature has been burgeoning very rapidly. To get a better understanding of RWD, Makady et al. (2017) conducted a literature review of PubMed, covering the period January 1, 2005, up to their last day of the search in December 31, 2016, spanning 11 years. Their initial PubMed search yielded 496 hits, whereas an additional search of the gray literature yielded 66 hits. The growth and interest in RWD and RWE have been very steep within the last few years. My own search of Elsevier's SCOPUS database on August 8, 2019, using the search term "real world data" on "abstract, title, or keywords" resulted in 15,297 hits of which 1,975 were in the subject area subgrouped as "medicine." When "real world evidence" was used instead as the search term, there were 901 hits with 801 in the subject area "medicine." Similarly, when I searched PubMed, "real world data" yielded 2,705 hits and "real world evidence" yielded 871 hits. This rapid growth in the scientific literature in just a few years clearly indicates significant and heightened interest of stakeholders on the topic, and it portrays a healthy growth in the research landscape of RWD and RWE. This is not surprising because the theoretical potential for financial savings through RWE-based medical product evaluations is substantial in an industry that spent $22.4 billion on phase 3 and phase 4 clinical trials in 2011 with an estimated total cost of R&D for a single drug at $2.9 billion (Bartlett et al. 2019).

Because quality of evidence is affected not only by appropriateness of statistical analyses but also, importantly, by quality of data and degree of representation of a patient population of interest, it will be necessary to explicitly define and describe RWD whenever evidence is generated and presented from such data. This is particularly important because RWD varies greatly. RWD can originate from a variety of sources, each with its own associated inherent biases and quality issues arising from measurement errors, all of which must be taken into consideration when evidence is generated from such data to inform health-related decisions that affect patients. Makady et al. (2017) conducted a review of definitions of RWD based on the published literature and their own stakeholder interviews. They concluded that, "a significant number of authors and stakeholders do not have an official, institutional definition for RWD," nor have they adopted definitions developed by societies and expert working groups such as the International Society for Pharmacoeconomics and Outcomes Research (ISPOR) and the Association of the British Pharmaceutical Industry (ABPI). Because the sources and types of RWD vary, any attempt to derive a single, all-encompassing definition of RWD can only be generic at best. One such generic and early definition of RWD can be traced to an ISPOR Task Force more than a decade ago, which simply defined it as "data used for decision-making that are not collected in conventional randomized clinical trials" (Bate 2016).

Based on their stakeholder interviews, Makady et al. (2017) stated that, "all stakeholders conceded data generated by RCTs are not RWD." This finding also agrees with a recent industry perspective presented by Khosla et al. (2018): "RWE is derived from the analysis of data collected from a healthcare setting, outside the context of prescriptive RCTs." According to Makady et al. (2017), RWD can be categorized into two sources: (1) data from sources such as claims databases and registries and (2) from study designs that generate RWD, such as observational studies and pragmatic clinical trials. Examples of RWD that emerged from their interviews of stakeholders included any health record information not collected as part of RCT, observational data collected without blinding and specific inclusion/exclusion criteria, data generated from non-controlled settings without random assignments, and data collected from routine clinical practice. Irrespective of the different sources of RWD, different qualities of evidence from such data may be acceptable for different purposes depending on whether they are "fit-for-purpose" or not to answer specific research questions of interest, or to make practical decisions. The phrase fit-for-purpose implies different tolerance levels for erroneous conclusions that can lead to incorrect decisions which, in turn, will be based on tolerance levels for different risk-benefit/cost-benefit scenarios. Khosla et al. (2018) underscored that all phases of medicine development ranging from pre-clinical to phase 4 and commercialization can benefit from RWD/RWE, such as with applications in shaping target product profile, designing phase 3 studies, achieving registration/approval, achieving access and reimbursement, and maintaining access and demonstrating continued value. Again, it is important to emphasize that each of these applications can have its own acceptable tolerance level for probability of obtaining correct evidence to support the decision-making process.

2.2 Why Is RWD Important?

To understand why RWD are important, we must begin by asking why RCTs alone do not provide adequate clinical evidence for treating patients optimally. RCTs are highly controlled experiments conducted to test specific hypotheses of treatment efficacy of a new investigational therapy (NIT) on an indication by randomizing treatments and carefully monitoring patients' adherence to study protocols. Evidence gathered from RCTs is considered the "gold standard" for assessing treatment efficacy of an NIT for a pathological indication when compared with either a standard of care (SOC) if another therapeutic product exists, or to a placebo if no other therapy exists. Randomization of treatments, blinding of study investigators and participants, and pre-specification of study protocol and statistical analysis plans (SAPs) are all necessary conditions for RCTs to be valid. Such study designs emerged in the second half of the twentieth century as the "methodological gold standard" for development and approval of new medicines, medical devices, and medical technologies (Rosemann 2019). Because RCTs are carefully controlled experiments, it becomes a practical necessity to constrain study design criteria and limit patient enrollment in such studies by using carefully chosen, strict inclusion/exclusion criteria.

This practical limitation in designing RCTs constitutes the first of two main shortcomings in evidence gathered from such studies. As RCTs are generally conducted with restricted samples of patients, they often do not represent adequately the broader patient populations who are seen in clinics. Figure 2.1 uses hypothetical data to illustrate potential bias and inadequate representation that can be encountered in data from an RCT. The two types of data displayed in the figure can be imagined as a Venn diagram in which the RCT data will be a nested smaller circle inside a larger circle that represents the RWD. The sample means and sample variances in the RCT and RWS data can be considerably different. As the RWD in Figure 2.1 show

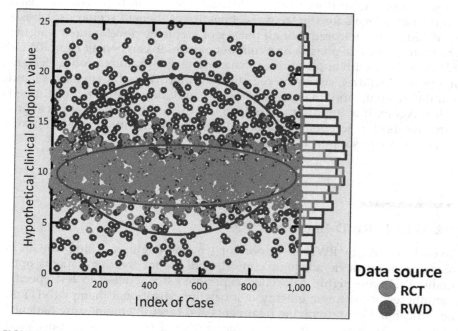

Data source
● RCT
● RWD

FIGURE 2.1
A hypothetical example of a primary clinical endpoint measured after treatment of 1000 patients enrolled in a randomized controlled trial (RCT), and 1000 patients who are treated in clinics representing the realworld data (RWD). The ellipses denote cases within one standard deviation of the mean for each data type. The right side of the figure displays histograms associated with the hypothetical data. The arithmetic average and standard deviation for the RCT data are 9.9, and 1.93, respectively. The arithmetic average and standard deviation for RWD are 11.7 and 5.79, respectively. These values correspond to coefficients of variation of 20 and 50% for RCT and RWD, respectively. Although the data are hypothetical, they portray realistic scenarios that could be encountered in the real world. Author's perspectives on why such differences should be considered important are further discussed in the text.

greater variation in the clinical endpoint of interest, extrapolation of efficacy inferences from the RCT data may lead to inflated overly optimistic expectations of patient benefits in the clinic. Clinical treatment decisions based on such inflated expectations may negatively impact some patients more than others. In Figure 2.1, the average value of the clinical endpoint measure in the RCT data is lower (mean of 9.9) than in the RWD (mean of 11.7). With an assumption that the better controlled RCT has resulted in a more optimistic outcome, values high on the Y-axis (for example, >15) in the RWD can be assumed to represent patients who will not benefit from the treatment. Unless RWD is collected and analyzed to generate RWE, such knowledge of the real world, especially deviations from results obtained in RCT, will remain largely unknown.

One way to obtain and contrast evidence of likely benefit to an individual patient (the essence of personalized medicine) between an RCT and RWD will be by pre-specifying in the study design what is a minimum clinically meaningful impact (MCMI) on an individual patient (for example, a cutoff in change from baseline value in a patient's clinical endpoint measure after undergoing treatment), and then to calculate the proportion of patients who attain such MCMI in RCT versus RWD. I have discussed such a perspective previously and have argued that if data showing proportion of patients on a treatment who attain MCMI are available, clinical decision-aiding questions can be answered objectively via an easily interpretable probabilistic scale (Khatry 2018a). Thus, all stakeholders involved in an individual patient's care (including the patient) will be able to obtain understandable answers to simple questions such as (see Khatry 2018a, for an extended discussion) (1) what is the probability that the patient will respond to treatment A, (2) what is the percentage point difference in likely response to treatment A (e.g., NIT) versus B (SOC), (3) what is the risk of not responding to treatment B compared with A, (4) what are the odds that treatment A will be better in eliciting response than treatment B, or (5) what is the probability that treatment A will be more efficacious for the patient than treatment B? In another related publication, I have demonstrated how clinical trial simulations of enrichment designs with different diagnostic accuracy criteria and clinical efficacy criteria can be used to plan for studies that will estimate probabilities of attaining evidence of both a medicine's improved efficacy over another treatment as well as evidence of its clinical effectiveness on how likely it will be to benefit an individual patient in a clinic (Khatry 2018b). RWD can greatly aid in conducting such simulations.

In the same vein, in his highly-cited essay titled, "Why Most Clinical Research Is Not Useful," Ioannidis (2016) has argued that "studying treatment effects under idealized clinical trial conditions is attractive, but questions then remain over the generalizability of the findings to real-life circumstances." This was similarly communicated earlier by Cole and Stuart (2010) who argued that RCTs typically provide stronger internal validity than observational study designs, but that they remain susceptible to a lack of external validity. It is important to note here a very important qualification of "randomization." Although randomization is used in clinical trials to randomly allocate treatments to individual patients, there is no randomization scheme implemented per se to sample clinical patients who are randomly selected to accurately represent the patient population of interest. Thus, RCTs constitute non-probability samples of patients and have similar limitations of generalizability as do convenience sampling, purposive sampling, quota sampling, respondent-driven sampling, and so forth. A relevant discussion of examples and limitations of various probability and non-probability sampling schemes can be found in the first published (of four planned) United States (U.S.) Food and Drug Administration (FDA) guidance on patient-focused drug development (FDA 2018).

The second shortcoming of evidence generated from RCTs also has to do with the propensity for "bias." In addition to potential bias in RCTs conducted with non-probability samples that often may not adequately represent the real-world clinical populations of interest, it is important to remember that biases also can occur because randomization in studies is carried out before study interventions. The goal of bias control in an RCT can be seriously undermined by events that occur after the randomization has been implemented at study start, such as from treatment discontinuation or switching of medicines by patients, poor adherence to treatment regimen, use of rescue medication, death of study participant, or missing data that may arise from any other cause. This is the reason regulatory agencies such as the European Medicines Agency (EMA) and the FDA are interested in potential use of "estimands" that require pre-specification of how intercurrent events will be accounted for in planned statistical analyses. In ICH E9 (R1), an addendum to the established guideline on statistical principles for clinical trials (ICH E9), Section A.1. (Purpose and Scope) specifically states (European Medicines Agency 2017):

> Randomized trials are expected to be free from baseline confounding but, in trials as in clinical practice, certain events will occur that complicate the description and interpretation of treatment effects. In this addendum, these are denoted as intercurrent events and include, among others, use of an alternative treatment (e.g. a rescue medication, a medication prohibited by the protocol or a subsequent line of therapy), discontinuation of treatment, treatment switching and terminal events such as, in some circumstances, death.

Thus, an important distinction to note here is that RCTs provide evidence of average clinical efficacy of an NIT in relatively narrowly defined non-probability study samples, whereas RWSs provide evidence of effectiveness of the therapy in broader patient groups that frequent clinical practices (Roland and Torgerson 1998; Khatry 2018a).

2.3 For What Purposes Can RWD Be Useful?

Khosla et al. (2018) have summarized potential uses of RWE from RWD, which spans the drug-discovery, product development, and commercialization spectrum for answering important questions, such as ones related to disease epidemiology and unmet medical need, patient pathways from diagnosis through treatments, patient population characteristics, feasibility of clinical trial protocols, safety and effectiveness in clinical applications, and product use in the real world. They postulate that such evidence can be used for purposes of shaping target product profile, designing pivotal phase 3 studies, achieving registration/approval, achieving access and reimbursement, and maintaining access while demonstrating continued value. Similarly, Bate (2016) provided examples of insight-generating potential uses of RWD at various stages of the drug development life cycle by asking these specific questions:

1. How many people suffer from the condition and also have comorbidities x and y, or what drugs are currently used in the treatment of a condition and to what extent are clinical guidelines being followed (discovery phase)?

2. Given efficacy and tolerability results from early trials how might current treatment pathways be affected by new drug, or how costly are specific areas of unmet need that a drug with such target product profile might address (early development phase)?

3. For the purpose of designing phase 3 trials what underlying rates of adverse events would be reasonable expectations in trial populations, or how can eligibility criteria in phase 3 protocols be modified to reduce recruitment problems (late development phase)?

4. What are likely budget impacts of introducing a new drug across different patient segments, or what potential safety issues might be seen with early use of the drug in practice (registration/market access phase)?

5. How can a large clinical trial using electronic medical records be run to show relative effectiveness of drug, or in which patient groups do drug compliance issues arise?

Clearly, potential applications of RWD to generate meaningful RWE are broad ranging, and I envision their potential utility spanning the entire biopharmaceutical R&D continuum starting from drug discovery projects all the way through to product life cycle management.

2.4 What Study Designs and Statistical Methods Will Be Necessary to Ensure High-Quality RWE?

Figure 2.2 illustrates similarities and important differences between a typical RCT and an RWS. The temporal flow of the two types of studies are illustrated by the arrows linking the sequentially arranged boxes. Both types of studies start out similarly with research questions of interest related to a drug's impact. The fifth and sixth sequential boxes are also similar between the two study types and denote data analyses and result-gathering steps. Sequential boxes two, three, and four show important differences between the two study types. The sequence in RCT begins with study design and writing of study protocol and prespecified SAP, followed by study site selection with randomized enrollment of patients, and then by prospective data collection. This sequence is altered in RWS. The sequence in RWS starts with retrospective selection of RWD, followed by study design and writing of study protocol and prespecified SAP, and then bias reduction by using propensity scores in lieu of randomization. The last set of boxes in Figure 2.1 denote what kind of primary evidence is generated from the two study designs. RCTs generate evidence of drug efficacy. RWSs generate RWE of the clinical effectiveness of a drug. Interestingly, a framework to link these two types of studies has been recently proposed by Selker et al. (2019). These authors propose what they called "efficacy-to-effectiveness (E2E) trials," in which positive outcomes from efficacy trials are transitioned seamlessly to an effectiveness trial component to efficiently yield evidence of both a drug's efficacy and its clinical effectiveness. Additional variations proposed by Selker et al. (2019) include simultaneously addressing efficacy and effectiveness in an "efficacy and effectiveness too (EE2)" trial and hybrids of the E2E and EE2 approaches with different degrees of overlap of the two components.

Along with evidence of drug efficacy and clinical effectiveness, RWSs can generate additional important types of evidence that can be used across the drug discovery and product life cycle management continuum. As previously stated, quality of RWE will depend on how fit-for-purpose applications are designated and users' willingness to tolerate different magnitudes of

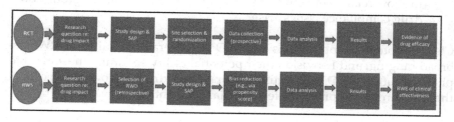

FIGURE 2.2
Similarities and differences in how clinical evidences are collected and how the evidences themselves differ between a randomized controlled trial (RCT) and real-world study (RWS). Abbreviations: statistical analysis plan (SAP); real world evidence (RWE).

error in risking potential erroneous conclusions that may lead to subsequent incorrect decision in applications. Error tolerance levels might be set higher for sponsors' internal decision-making purposes such as in drug discovery or early development applications, but error tolerance requirements will need to be made more stringent in late-stage drug development, or for presentation to external stakeholders such as regulators, prescribers, payers, and key opinion leaders (KOLs) who have influential roles in developing clinical guidelines. Therefore, optimal designs of RWSs and the statistical methods of analyses will depend on both the attributes of RWD and the specific objectives of and audiences for the studies.

An ISPOR Task Force was commissioned in 2007 to review and recommend statistical control of confounding in non-randomized studies. The task force—which drew members from industry, academia and government, and from across Europe, Canada, and the United States with members' experience in medicine, epidemiology, biostatistics, public health, health economics, and pharmacy sciences—developed a report that specifically addressed methods to improve causal inference of treatment effects for non-randomized studies (Johnson et al. 2009). Specific recommendations were made for general analytic techniques and best practices that included use of stratification analysis before multivariable modeling, multivariable regressions including model performance and diagnostic testing, propensity scoring, instrumental variable, and structural modeling techniques that included marginal structural models and sensitivity analyses. The task force's recommendations have been described in detail by Johnson et al. (2009), and more recently as abbreviated good practice recommendations by Berger et al. (2017).

Another excellent description of methods, cautions, and recommendations for building reliable evidence from RWD is presented by Corrao (2013) and Corrao and Cantarutti (2018). Corrao (2013) provided a methodological framework for researchers that describes (1) strategies for sampling within a large cohort as an alternative to analyzing the full cohort, (2) methods for controlling outcome and exposure misclassifications, (3) techniques that take into account both measured and unmeasured confounders, (4) specific considerations regarding random uncertainty in the framework of observational studies based on healthcare utilization data, and (5) recommendations for good research practice.

The regulatory agencies in the United States and Europe are actively engaging in, and are supportive of, potential use of RWD to generate RWE because they believe that RWE could potentially expedite their regulatory decision-making. As part of the initiatives created by the 21st Century Cures Act, the FDA released the first patient-focused drug development draft guideline in June 2018, and the second of four planned draft guidelines in October 2019 (FDA 2018, 2019). The second document is aimed at guiding sponsors to identify what is most important to patients concerning their experience with burden of disease and treatments. The release of the second draft guideline by the FDA coincided with the publication of a new perspective article on patient engagement, which was jointly coauthored by FDA and EMA officials and published in the journal *Nature Reviews Drug Discovery* (Calvert et al. 2019). In another recent publication coauthored by some European regulators, Eichler et al. 2020 recommended the use of transparent, collaborative platforms such as EMA's methods qualification procedure or similar procedures offered by the FDA and other public bodies. They caution that to make novel analytical methods acceptable for regulators and other decision makers, testing and validation will be required in broadly the same way as one would evaluate a new drug: "prospectively, well-controlled and according to pre-agreed plan." Extensive details with tables and charts of study designs, data limitations, and statistical analyses methods for utilizing RWD to generate RWE are provided in the regulatory draft guidelines and the published perspective papers authored by the European and U.S. regulators (interested readers are specifically referred to FDA 2018, 2019, Calvert et al. 2019, and Eichler et al. 2020).

2.5 Some Application Examples

I will now use some examples to illustrate potential applications of RWE. I will begin with a hypothetical and very simple example from severe asthma. Between 5% and 10% of patients with asthma experience difficult asthma (i.e., with poor disease control despite treatment with high-dose inhaled corticosteroids and long-acting β-agonists), and such severe asthma is complex and heterogenous (Denton et al. 2019). Three anti-eosinophilic biologics (GSK's mepolizumab, Teva Pharmaceutical's reslizumab, and AstraZeneca's benralizumab) were recently approved by regulators for marketing, and these drugs are potentially available in the clinic to treat severe asthmatics. Let us assume Figure 2.3 shows dot density distributions of the asthma

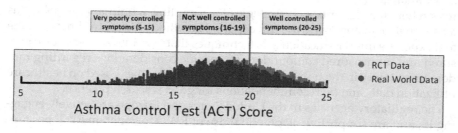

FIGURE 2.3
A hypothetical example of ACT scores of 1000 severe asthma patients each from RCT and RWD after treatment with a new therapy. The arithmetic mean, standard deviation, and median for RCT are 18.8, 2.9, and 18.9, respectively. The arithmetic mean, standard deviation, and median for RWD are 17.8, 2.9, and 17.9, respectively. 34.1% (341/1000) patients in the RCT have well-controlled asthma after receiving a new treatment, whereas only 22.1% (221/1000) patients in the RWD have well-controlled asthma after receiving a new treatment. Thus, in the RCT, 54% more patients are well-controlled after the treatment than in data collected from real-world clinical practice. Is this evidence of difference between RCT and clinical practice important to know by stakeholders? Author's perspectives are further discussed in the text.

control test (ACT) scores, which is a primary clinical endpoint for asthma quality of control, measured in individual asthma patients after treatment by one of those three drugs in an RCT and in the clinic. The ACT is a validated 5-item, patient-completed measure of asthma control with a recall period of 4 weeks, and an ACT score ≤19 is useful for identifying patients with poorly controlled asthma as defined by the Global Initiative for Asthma (GINA) (Thomas et al. 2009). The means, medians, and standard deviations of the scores in the hypothetical RCT data and the RWD are not very different between RCT and RWD (see Figure 2.3 legend), but there is a shift to the right toward higher scores in the distribution of the RCT data. What useful clinical evidence can be generated from these two data sets, and do they provide meaningful decision-aiding information to different stakeholders (for example, to patients, prescribers, and payers) for deciding whether to or not to use the drug in the clinic?

One important and potentially clinically useful evidence that can be extracted from the hypothetical data displayed in Figure 2.3 is that 34.1% (341/1000) patients in the RCT have well-controlled asthma after receiving a new treatment, whereas only 22.1% (221/1000) patients in the RWD have well-controlled asthma after receiving the very same new treatment in a real-world setting. Thus, if attainment of well-controlled asthma (ACT score >19) is a clinical treatment goal, the probability that a patient who visits a real-world clinic to receive the treatment will meet that goal is 22%, whereas the RCT data indicated it should be 34%. Is this evidence of clinical effectiveness in the real world, which is 54% lower for an individual patient than would be expected from the RCT results, important to know and useful for making decision on whether to or not to adopt the treatment? Different patients, prescribers, and payers will have their own criteria on deciding whether this difference in RCT data versus the RWD is important. Additionally, this information will be used along with other clinically relevant information, such as whether alternate products are available or not for treatment, how evidence of clinical effectiveness differs among the products, what are the potential differences in costs and ease and frequency of applications such as subcutaneous vs. intravenous injections, and so forth. The key point here is that RWD allow such evidence to be generated for asking specific questions that can facilitate better-informed clinical decision-making.

Now let us look at some applications that generated RWE using RWD. Subsequent discussions below of evidence synthesized from RWD are extracted directly from my own first-hand experiences. As a former employee of AstraZeneca, I was involved in the development of an anti-eosinophilic biologic (anti-IL5rα mAb), benralizumab, to treat patients with severe asthma and chronic obstructive pulmonary disease (COPD). Benralizuamb is currently marketed worldwide as Fasenra for the treatment of severe asthma patients. While the pivotal phase 3 RCTs of benralizumab were being conducted, it was decided by AstraZeneca leadership that generating parallel RWE related to the "eosinophilic" disease itself, and how an anti-eosinophilic biologic could potentially benefit such patients, would be important for communicating scientific and clinical knowledge to stakeholders, and also potentially useful during commercialization if the phase 3 trials succeed and regulatory approval is obtained to market the drug. AstraZeneca signed an agreement with Kaiser Permanente in Southern California (KPSC) to use their large administrative RWD from their research warehouse to conduct specific studies. Trung Tran, an AstraZeneca colleague, and I collaborated with KPSC's Robert Zeiger and other investigators to generate meaningful RWE from their RWD, and we co-published seven peer-reviewed papers from the collaboration, which have provided valuable clinical insights related to severe asthma and COPD, and other potential clinical implications for using anti-eosinophilic treatments such as benralizumab.

The RWE synthesized from our carefully pre-specified and planned analyses of the KPSC RWD demonstrated the following clinically useful insights:

1. Population care management programs and clinical practice should consider measurement of the blood eosinophil count as an additional biologic marker to assist in the identification of persistent adult patients with asthma and with higher risk for future exacerbations and excessive short-acting β_2-agonist use (Zeiger et al. 2014).

2. Blood eosinophil counts of $300/mm^3$ or more in children with persistent asthma may identify children at increased risk for future asthma exacerbations, indicating a possible higher disease burden among those patients (Zeiger et al. 2015a).

3. Higher disease burden in high-risk, high-adherent patients suggests that healthcare organizations and clinicians need to target this subgroup with higher level step-care, more asthma specialist care, attention to relevant comorbidities, and judicious use of existing and novel new biologicals (Zeiger et al. 2015b).

4. There is a greater disease burden associated with elevated blood eosinophil levels in patients with persistent asthma (PA) who also have a COPD diagnosis code (AS-COPD), which suggests a common inflammatory component between AS-COPD and PA only (Zeiger et al. 2016).

5. Population care management programs in asthma need to identify chronic oral corticosteroid users to institute more intensive patient management and treatment (Zeiger et al. 2017).

6. GINA step-care level 4 or 5, frequent asthma exacerbations, excessive rescue bronchodilator use, and elevated blood eosinophil count are among the independent cost predictors associated with increased asthma-related total healthcare costs for adults aged 18 to 64 years with persistent asthma (Zeiger et al. 2018a).

7. To improve outcomes for patients with COPD, population care management programs and clinical practice could consider measurement

of blood eosinophil count to identify a phenotype with elevated blood eosinophils who might benefit with specific anti-inflammatory and anti-eosinophilic therapies (Zeiger et al. 2018b).

Clearly, these RWSs that analyzed the KPSC administrative data provided many clinically meaningful insights related to severe asthma, which included demonstration of blood eosinophil levels as important considerations in phenotyping asthma for targeted management in the clinic. Further corroboration of clinical evidence extracted from RWD on the importance of blood eosinophils in severe asthma was made by our separate analysis of an independent RWD, the National Health and Nutrition Examination Survey (NHANES). After analyzing the NHANES data, we reported that asthma patients with higher blood eosinophil counts experienced more asthma attacks than those with lower eosinophil counts (Tran et al. 2014).

Other examples of RWE generation from RWD are increasingly populating the literature. An often-cited example is the "Salford Lung Study (SLS)" (Bakerly et al. 2015). The SLS collected EHR data and assessed effectiveness and safety of fluticasone furoate in COPD patients in the United Kingdom. Seventy-five general practitioner clinics, 128 community pharmacies in Salford and South Manchester, and two hospitals participated in a 12-month, open-label, phase 3 study in which 2,799 patients were randomized 1:1 to a once-daily inhaled combination of fluticasone furoate 100 μg and vilanterol 25 μg, or to a continuation of their existing therapy. For a detailed discussion of the SLS case study, and another large observational study on amyotrophic lateral sclerosis (ALS) conducted by PatientsLikeMe, readers are referred to Khosla et al. (2018). In another recently-published review, Webster and Smith (2019) made a case for using RWE in chronic myeloid leukemia (CML). They reported that in CML, RWE has informed early treatment milestones and has provided a window into patient perspectives regarding treatment, and that such information from the real world will help clinicians to better optimize treatments. Thus, RWD and RWE are already aiding clinical decisions and generating insights that are relevant across the healthcare ecosystem.

2.6 Summary

Acceleration in the use of RWD to generate RWE can be expected to continue with new developments in technology and advancements in computer-aided analytics. However, the reliability and validity of the evidence generated from RWD must be assured through strict adherence to data quality and the fundamental principles of the "scientific method of inquiry," which include well-designed studies, pre-specified SAPs, and independent validations of key findings. More data are not necessarily better, and potential outcomes arising from "garbage-in-garbage-out (GIGO)" situations must be carefully avoided. Although there can be variations in guidelines on cautions and recommendations in the generation of RWE from RWD, the recommendations for good procedural practices provided by the ISPOR-ISPE Special Task Force on RWE in healthcare decision-making (Berger et al. 2017) are sound. The ISPOR-ISPE task force has recommended the following seven criteria: (1) *a priori*, determine that a study is exploratory or a hypothesis evaluating treatment effectiveness (HETE); (2) post a HETE study protocol and SAP on a public study registration site before conducting data analysis; (3) publish HETE study results with attestation to conformance and/or deviation from study protocol and pre-specified SAP; (4) enable transparency so that other researchers can replicate study findings; (5) validate study findings on independent data; (6) address methodological criticisms of study after publication; and (7) include key stakeholders in designing, conducting, and disseminating HETE studies. The many types of exploratory versus HETE spectrum of evidence, which can be generated from RWD, could have applications across the entire drug-discovery/development through the product life cycle management continuum, and individual studies can be designed with different error tolerance levels based on pre-determined fit-for-purpose applications.

References

Bakerly, N.D., Woodcock, A., New, J.P., Gibson, J.M., Wu, W., Leather, D., and Vestbo, J. 2015. The Salford Lung Study protocol: a pragmatic, randomized phase III real-world effectiveness trial in chronic obstructive pulmonary disease. *Respiratory Research*, 16, 101. DOI 10.1186/s12931-015-0267-6.

Bartlett, V.L., Dhruva, S.S., Shah, N.D., Ryan, P., and Ross, J.S. 2019. Feasibility of using real-world data to replicate clinical trial evidence. *JAMA Network Open*, 2(10), e1912869. doi:10.1001/jamanetworkopen.2019.12869.

Bate, A. 2016. Designing and incorporating a real world data approach to international drug development and use: what the UK offers. *Drug Discovery Today*, 21(3), 400–405.

Berger, M.L., Sox, H., Eillke, R.J., Brixner, D.L., Eichler, H.-G., Goettsch, W., Madigan, D., Makady, A., Schneeweiss, S., Tarricone, R., Wang, S.W., Watkins, J., and Mullins, C.D. 2017. Good practices for real-world data studies of treatment and/or comparative effectiveness: Recommendations from the joint ISPOR-ISPE Special Task Force on real-world evidence in health care decision making. *Pharmacoepidemiology and Drug Safety*, 26, 1033–1039.

Calvert, M.J., O'Connor, D.J., and Basch, E.M. 2019. Harnessing the patient voice in real-world evidence: the essential role of patient-reported outcomes. *Nature Reviews Drug Discovery*, 18, 731–732.

Cole, S.R. and Stuart, E.A. 2010. Generalizing evidence from randomized clinical trials to target populations: The ACTG 320 Trial. *American Journal of Epidemiology*, 172, 107–115.

Corrao, G. 2013. Building reliable evidence from real-world data: methods, cautiousness and recommendations. *Epidemiology Biostatistics and Public Health*, 10(3), e8981-1–e8981-40.

Corrao, G., and Cantarutti, A. 2018. Building reliable evidence from real-world data: Needs, methods, cautiousness and recommendations. *Pulmonary Pharmacology & Therapeutics*, 53, 61–67.

Denton, E., Hore-Lacy, F., Radhakrishna, N., Gilbert, A., Tay, T., Lee, J., Dabschek, E., Harvey, E.S., Bulathsinhala, L., Fingleton, J., Price, D., Gibson, P., O'hehir, R., and Hew, M. 2019. Severe asthma global evaluation (SAGE): An electronic platform for severe asthma. *Journal of Allergy and Clinical Immunology in Practice*, 7(5), 1440–1449.

Eichler, H.-G., Koenig, F., Arlett, P., Enzmann, H., Humphreys, A., Petavy, F., Schwarzer-Daum, B., Sepodes, B., Vamvakas, S., and Rasi, G. 2020. Are novel, non-randomised analytic methods fit for decision-making? The need for prospective, controlled and transparent validation. *Clinical Pharmacology & Therapeutics*, 107(4), 773–779.

European Medicines Agency. 2017. ICH E9 (R1) Addendum on Estimands and Sensitivity Analysis in Clinical Trials to the Guideline On Statistical Principles For Clinical Trials. Step 2b. https://www.ema.europa.eu/en/documents/scientific-guideline/draft-ich-e9-r1-addendum-estimands-sensitivity-analysis-clinical-trials-guideline-statistical_en.pdf (accessed on June 9, 2020).

Food and Drug Administration. 2018. Patient-Focused Drug Development: Collecting Comprehensive and Representative Input. Guidance for industry, Food and Drug Administration staff and other stakeholders. Draft Guidance. https://www.federalregister.gov/documents/2018/06/13/2018-12636/patient-focused-drug-development-collecting-comprehensive-and-representative-input-draft-guidance (accessed on June 9, 2020).

Food and Drug Administration. 2019. Patient-Focused Drug Development: Methods to Identify What Is Important to Patients. Guidance for Industry, Food and Drug Administration Staff and Other Stakeholders. Draft Guidance (accessed on June 9, 2020).

Ford, I. and Norrie, J. 2016. Pragmatic trials. *The New England Journal of Medicine*, 375, 454–463.

Godwin, M., Ruhland, L., Casson, I., MacDonald, S., Delva, D., Birtwhistle, R., Lam, M., and Seguin, R. 2003. Pragmatic controlled clinical trials in primary care: the struggle between external and internal validity. *BMC Medical Research Methodology*, 3(28), 7.

Ioannidis, J.P.A. 2016. Why most clinical research is not useful. *PLoS Medicine*, 13(6), e1002049. doi:10.1371/journal pmed. 1002049.

Irving, E., van den Bor, R., Welsing, P., Walsh, V., Alfonso-Cristancho, R., Harvey, C., Garman, N., Grobbee, D.E., and GetReal Work Package 3. 2017. Series: Pragmatic trials and real world evidence: Paper 7. Safety, quality and monitoring. *Journal of Clinical Epidemiology*, 91, 6–12.

Johnson, M.L., Crown, W., Martin, B.C., Dormuth, C.R., and Eiebert, U. 2009. Good research practices for comparative effectiveness research: Analytic methods to improve causal inference from nonrandomized studies of treatment effects using secondary data sources: The ISPOR Good Research Practices for Retrospective Database Analysis Task Force Report—Part III. *Value in Health*, 12(8), 1062–1073.

Kalkman, S., van Thiel, G.J.M.W., Zuidgeest, M.G.P., Goetz, I., Pfeiffer, B.M., Grobbee, D.E., van Delden, J.J.M., and Work Package 3 of the IMI GetReal consortium. 2017.

Series: Pragmatic trials and real world evidence: Paper 4. Informed consent. *Journal of Clinical Epidemiology*, 89, 181–187.

Khatry, D.B. 2018a. Demonstrating efficacy and effectiveness in clinical studies with recurrent event as primary endpoint: A simulation example of COPD. *Journal of Comparative Effectiveness Research*, 7 (10), 935–945.

Khatry, D.B. 2018b. Precision medicine in clinical practice. *Personalized Medicine*, 15(5), 413–417.

Khosla, S., White, R., Medina, J., Ouwens, M., Emmas, C., Koder, T., Male, G,. and Leonard, S. 2018. Real world evidence (RWE) – a disruptive innovation or the quiet evolution of medical evidence generation? *F1000Research* 7, 1111. DOI: https://doi.org/10.12688/f1000research13585.2.

Makady, A., de Boer, A., Hilege, H., Klungel, O., Goettsch, W., and GetReal Work Package 1. 2017. What is real-world data? A review of definitions based on literature and stakeholder interviews. *Value in Health*, 20, 858–865.

Meinecke, A.-K., Welsing, P., Kafatos, G., Burke, D., Trelle, S., Kubin, M., Nachbaur, G., Egger, M., Zuidgeest, M., and Work package 3 of the GetReal consortium. 2017. Series: Pragmatic trials and real world evidence: Paper 8. Data collection and management. *Journal of Clinical Epidemiology*, 91, 13–22.

Mutz, D.C. 2011. *Population-Based Survey Experiments*. Princeton, NJ: Princeton University Press.

Rengerink, K.O., Kalkman, S., Collier, S., Ciaglia, A., Worsley, S.D., Lightbourne, A., Eckert, L., Groenwold, R.H.H., Grobbee, D.E., Irving, E.A., and Work Package 3 of the GetReal consortium. 2017. Series: Pragmatic trials and real world evidence: Paper 3. Patient selection challenges and consequences. *Journal of Clinical Epidemiology*, 89, 173–180.

Roland, M. and Torgerson, D.J. 1998. Understanding controlled trials: What are pragmatic trials? *BMJ*, 316, 285.

Rosemann, A. 2019. After-standardizing clinical trials: The gold standard in the crossfire. *Science as Culture*, 29(2), 125–148.

Selker, H.P., Eichler, H.-G., Stockbridge, N.L., McElwee, N.E., Dere, W.H., Cohen, T., Erban, J.K., Seyfert-Margolis, V.L., Honig, P.K., Kaitin, K.I., Oye, K.A., and D'Agostino Sr, R.B. 2019. Efficacy and effectiveness too trials: Clinical trial designs to generate evidence on efficacy and on effectiveness in wide practice. *Clinical Pharmacology & Therapeutics*, 105(4), 857–866.

Tran, T.N., Khatry, D.B., Ke, X., Ward, C.K., and Gossage, D. 2014. High blood eosinophil count is associated with more frequent asthma attacks in asthma patients. *Annals of Allergy, Asthma & Immunology*, 113, 19–24.

Thomas, M., Kay, S., Pike, J., Williams, A., Rosenzweig, J.R.C., Hillyer, E.V., and Price, D. 2009. The Asthma Control Test™ (ACT) as a predictor of GINA guideline-defined asthma control: analysis of a multinational cross-sectional survey. *Primary Care Respiratory Journal*, 18(1), 41–49.

Webster, J. and Smith, B.D. 2019. The case for real-world evidence in the future of clinical research on chronic myeloid leukemia. *Clinical Therapeutics*, 41(2), 336–349.

Welsing, P.M., Rengerink, K.O., Collier, S., Eckert, L., van Smeden, M., Ciaglia, A., Nachbaur, G., Trelle, S., Taylor, A.J., Egger, M., Goetz, I., and Work Package 3 of the GetReal consortium. 2017. Series: Pragmatic trials and real world evidence: Paper 6. Outcome measures in the real world. *Journal of Clinical Epidemiology*, 90, 99–107.

Worsley, S.D., Rengerink, K.O., Irving, E., Lejeune, S., Mol, K., Collier, S., Groenwold, R.H.H., Enters-Weijnen, C., Egger, M., Rhodes, T., and GetReal Work Package 3. 2017.

Series: Pragmatic trials and real world evidence: Paper 2. Setting, sites, and investigator selection. *Journal of Clinical Epidemiology*, 88, 14–20.

Zeiger, R.S., Schatz, M., Li, Q., Chen, W., Khatry, D.B., Gossage, D., and Tran, T.N. 2014. High blood eosinophil count is a risk factor for future asthma exacerbations in adult persistent asthma. *Journal of Allergy and Clinical Immunology in Practice*, 2(6), 741–750.

Zeiger, R.S., Schatz, M., Li, Q., Chen, W., Khatry, D.B., Gossage, D., and Tran, T.N. 2015a. The association of blood eosinophil counts to future asthma exacerbations in children with persistent asthma. *Journal of Allergy and Clinical Immunology in Practice*, 3(2), 283–287.e4.

Zeiger, R.S., Schatz, M., Li, Q., Chen, W., Khatry, D.B., and Tran, T.N. 2015b Adherent uncontrolled adult persistent asthma: characteristics and asthma outcomes. *Journal of Allergy and Clinical Immunology in Practice*, 3 (6), 986–990.e2.

Zeiger, R.S., Schatz, M., Li, Q., Chen, W., Khatry, D.B., and Tran, T.N. 2016. Characteristics and outcomes of HEDIS-defined asthma patients with COPD diagnostic coding. *Journal of Allergy and Clinical Immunology in Practice*, 4(2), 273–283.

Zeiger, R.S., Schatz, M., Li, Q., Chen, W., Khatry, D.B., and Tran, T.N. 2017. Burden of oral corticosteroid use by adults with persistent asthma. *Journal of Allergy and Clinical Immunology in Practice*, 5 (4), 1050–1060.e9.

Zeiger, R.S., Tran, T.N., Schatz, M., Li, Q., Chen, W., Khatry, D.B., Davis, J., and Kawatkar, A.A. 2018a. Drivers of health care costs for adults with persistent asthma. *Journal of Allergy and Clinical Immunology in Practice*, 6(1), 265–268.e4.

Zeiger, R.S., Tran, T.N., Butler, R.K., Schatz, M., Qiaowu Li, Q., Khatry, D.B., Martin, U., Kawatkar, A.A., and Chen, W. 2018b. Relationship of blood eosinophil counts to COPD exacerbations. *Journal of Allergy and Clinical Immunology in Practice*, 6(3), 944–954.e5.

Zuidgeest, M.G.P., Goetz, I., Groenwold, R.H.H., Irving, E., van Thiel, G.J.M.W., Grobbee, D.E., and GetReal Work Package 3. 2017a. Series: Pragmatic trials and real world evidence: Paper 1. Introduction. *Journal of Clinical Epidemiology*, 88, 7–13.

Zuidgeest, M.G.P., Welsing, P.M.J., van Thiel, G.J.M.W., Ciaglia, A., Alfonso-Cristancho, R., Eckert, L., Eijkemans, M.J.C., Egger, M., and WP3 of the GetReal consortium. 2017b. Series: Pragmatic trials and real world evidence: Paper 5. Usual care and real life comparators. *Journal of Clinical Epidemiology*, 90, 92–98.

3

Real-World Evidence from Population-Based Cancer Registry Data

Binbing Yu

3.1 Introduction

The war against cancer is a continual effort to find a cure [1, 2]. It is widely considered a priority for the society and government as cancer remains a major cause of death. Throughout the world, about 14 million new cancer cases and 8 million cancer deaths occur each year and cancer burden increases as the population ages. Despite the tremendous progress in cancer research and breakthroughs in cancer treatments, including targeted therapies and the recent emergence of cancer immunotherapies, many cancers still remain a huge challenge, and the poor survival prognosis indicates tremendous unmet patients' needs. The regulatory approval of new cancer drugs is built on a benefit-risk assessment. However, with the advances in genetic and other molecular and clinical subclassifications of cancers, the number of patients available for a specific clinical trial may be too few for a reliable evaluation of efficacy and safety. The traditional approaches to cancer drug development and approval may be complemented with real-world data (RWD) and real-world evidence (RWE) [3].

RWE refers to information and evidence gathered from data collected outside of the traditional clinical research setting. RWD can be found in disease registries, electronic health records (EHRs), insurance administration, and personal health devices. Traditionally, observational RWE is often derived and used in clinical epidemiological studies, in safety evaluation of medical products, and in post-marketing surveillance studies required by the regulatory agencies [4].

There are many benefits of using RWD in oncology drug development. Single-arm clinical trials are increasingly used in oncology when the comparison is made with historical controls, particularly when a large treatment effect is expected or randomized trials with placebo are not feasible or ethical [5]. The choice of the right comparator drug is critical when healthcare providers translate trial results into meaningful treatment scenarios. RWD can guide and inform pharmaceutical companies to select the most appropriate comparator, and RWD can provide evidence of the natural course of disease progression with and without medical interventions. Second, progression-free survival (PFS) and/or overall survival (OS) data are the most typical efficacy endpoints in drug development and evaluation. However, the efficacy evaluation is often based on clinical trials with limited study duration. Clinical trials usually provide limited information about long-term safety or quality of life data for the cancer treatment. Particularly health technology assessment (HTA) decision makers are often posed with limited clinical trial data at the time of drug approval. The need for comparative RWD to address the question about the long-term benefit and risk of a therapeutic agent is increasing when there is limited data from clinical trials, such as small cell lung cancer (SCLC).

The use of RWD to address clinical and policy-relevant questions that cannot be answered using data from clinical trials is generating increased interest [6]. In this chapter, we describe how to use RWD from the population-based cancer registry to evaluate the trends and burden of cancer and how to utilize the RWE to compare the long-term benefit of a particular cancer treatment. First, we describe the population-based cancer registry and introduce the most important measures of cancer burden based on the population-based registry data. We describe several statistical methods for analyzing the trends and pattern of cancer incidence, mortality, and survival. Using SCLC as an example, we describe how to combine the data from the clinical trial and the population-based cancer registry to extrapolate the long-term survival for the estimation and comparison of the expected life.

3.1.1 Population-Based Cancer Registry

Continuous, robust, and representative data and statistics on cancer occurrence are important to monitor the impact and trends of cancer, to identify public health priorities, and to evaluate the progress of cancer control programs in the society [2]. The main goal of population-based cancer registries is to provide such data by collecting information on all patients diagnosed with cancer in the general population. The first population-based cancer registries were created in 1929 in Germany. Now there are several hundred cancer registries that cover about 21% of the world population [7]. The data in a cancer registry are standardized according to international guidelines to ensure quality, completeness, and comparability. Originally, the role of cancer registries was limited to describe the burden, trends, and geographical comparisons of cancer. Gradually, many cancer registries expanded the data collection to include survival data to assess the overall efficacy of the cancer treatment. More recently, clinical variables, e.g., historical stages at diagnosis and certain molecular biomarkers, are included in the cancer registry to address the growing need for personalized healthcare and health disparity assessment. Currently, the Centers for Disease Control and Prevention (CDC) in the United States collects cancer data for 96% of the U.S. population through the National Program of Cancer Registries.

Cancer patients, healthcare providers, public health professionals, cancer researchers, and policy makers all need updated information about newly diagnosed cancer cases and deaths to better understand the impact and address the burden of cancer. Reliable estimates of the cancer burden and trends can provide a comprehensive picture of how the impact of cancer varies between geographic areas and changes temporarily. These cancer estimates provide input to the development of cancer control strategies. Increasingly, survival trends are also used to assess the efficacy of cancer strategies in reducing the impact of cancer over time. Incidence, survival, and mortality are the most popular measures in cancer epidemiology. They have been the principal measures to explore the causes and outcomes of cancer and to assess the effectiveness of cancer management programs. Cancer surveillance includes the monitoring of population levels and trends in incidence, survival, mortality, and prevalence of cancer. In addition, the factors that influence the cancer trends across the entire cancer control continuum, such as healthy populations at risk of cancer, new diagnosis of cancer, treatment of cancer, living with cancer, and dying of cancer or other causes, are also collected. For the analysis and interpretation of the cancer statistics collected by population-based cancer registries, a suite of statistical methodology has been developed by the U.S. National Cancer Institute (NCI) and other institutions throughout the world.

3.1.2 Cancer Incidence and Mortality Rates

Cancer incidence and mortality rates are essential population-based measures for public health and cancer control [8]. Cancer incidence is defined as how many people get a particular type of cancer. The crude incidence rate is often expressed as the number of cancer cases per 100,000 people in the general population because the crude rates are influenced by the underlying age distribution of the study cohort. Even if two cohorts have the same age-specific rates for each age group, the cohort with a relatively older population tends to have higher crude rates because incidence or death rates for most cancers increase with age. Naturally, the age distribution of a population can shift over time and may be different in different geographic regions. Adjusting the rates by age distribution removes the impact of different age distribution in the comparison of rates from different calendar years and different areas.

The age-adjusted incidence rate is most often computed using the direct method as it is the simplest and most straightforward method of standardization [9]. Suppose that the age is divided into I intervals, e.g., 5-year intervals up to age 79 and one interval for all ages greater than or equal to 80. Let d_i be the number of cancer cases in age interval i and n_i be the number of population in the midyear in age interval $i, i = 1, ..., I$. The age-specific incidence rate is calculated as

$$r_i = d_i / n_i, i = 1, ..., I. \tag{3.1}$$

The age-adjusted incidence rate is a weighted average of the age-specific incidence rates where the age-specific weights are the relative age proportion of the standard population. Let w_i be the proportion in age interval i in the standard population. The age-adjusted incidence rate (AAIR) is calculated as

$$AAIR = \sum_i w_i r_i = \sum_i w_i d_i / n_i. \tag{3.2}$$

Another less commonly used adjustment is the indirect standardization [9], which is useful when age-specific numbers of incidences are not available. Here we focus on the age-adjusted rate by direct standardization. The mortality is defined as the number of deaths due to a specific cancer of interest during a specific time period. The crude and age-adjusted mortality rates can be defined similarly as the incidence. Crude rates are helpful in determining the cancer burden and specific needs for cancer care for a given population, compared with another population, regardless of size.

Because cancer mortality is less influenced by the biases and inaccuracy of cancer diagnosis than survival and incidence, the mortality data derived from death certificates are often viewed as the ultimate indicator of cancer progress. However, the reported mortality data in cancer registries often lack information pertaining to the onset of disease, such as calendar year and age of diagnosis, cancer stage, and histological type at diagnosis. For example, SCLC has two subtypes, i.e., small cell carcinoma (about 90%) and combined small cell carcinoma (about 10%). Although it is not clear whether this division is clinically significant, it may be taken into account when therapy is considered. For the combined tumor type, SCLC may be mixed with a second histological component of NSCLC (large cell, adenocarcinoma, or squamous cell) and the relative balance of the subtypes within the tumor may shift after chemotherapy. It is not possible to estimate mortality trends for either of these subtypes of disease using U.S. mortality data because the histology of a cancer is not recorded on the death certificate. However, population-based cancer registries collect these types of data and allow the calculation of an incidence-based mortality (IBM) rate [10]. The IBM rate allows a partitioning of mortality by variables associated with the cancer diagnosis. IBM requires high-quality population-based cancer registry data and close follow-up of cancer patients for vital status including cause of death.

At a certain calendar year, let d_{ij} be the number of deaths for age group i and subgroup j, e.g., histological subtype, let n_i be the associated population, and w_i be the weight of age group i associated with a standard population, then the age-adjusted estimate of IBM rate for subgroup j is calculated as

$$IBM_j = \sum_i w_i d_{ij} / n_i.$$

The total estimate of the IBM rate is the sum of IBM across all level j of the factor, i.e.,

$$IBM = \sum_j IBM_j.$$

The total IBM rate may approximate the mortality rate based on the death certificate, but it will not equal it exactly. Mortality rates based on death certificates represent all of the deaths that occur within a certain geographical region, regardless of where the person lived when they were diagnosed with the disease. On the other hand, the IBM rate represents death certificates for everyone who was a resident of a registry catchment area when they were diagnosed with the cancer regardless of the location when they died. Usually, the bias of the IBM rate is relatively small. However, one should be cautious about possible lead-time bias in the IBM analysis [11]. The advantage of the IBM rate is that it can be used to partition the disease-specific mortality rates by factors associated with the disease at diagnosis.

3.1.3 Population-Based Cancer Survival

Cancer survival is one of the most important measures for monitoring and evaluating the effectiveness of cancer care. Due to improvements in cancer treatments and dissemination of early diagnosis techniques, there has been considerable progress against cancer. If diagnosed early and treated successfully, a proportion of patients may be cured for many types of cancer. The advantage of population-based survival analysis is that the results of such studies are representative of the entire population, a perspective which is vital for cancer control activities.

If the information on cause of death is reliable or recorded accurately. Then cause-specific survival analysis can be used to estimate the survival rate of cancer patients. The cancer-specific survival function $S(t)$ can be calculated by treating death due to other causes as censoring. However, in population-based cancer studies, cause of death may be either incorrectly identified or obtained from death certificates that are often inaccurately recorded [12]. For instance, it is not clear how to handle "autopsy only" cases and cases with unknown cause of death. As an alternative, relative survival [13] is often used as a measure of net survival (excess mortality) due to cancer under study. The relative survival is calculated as $S(t) = S_A(t)/S_E(t)$, where t is the survival time after the diagnosis of cancer; $S_A(t)$ is the observed OS rate for the cancer patient group; and $S_E(t)$ is the expected survival rate of a comparable group from the general population who are assumed to be practically free of the cancer of interest. The relative survival definition implies an additive hazards model, where the hazard of OS,

$$\lambda_A(t) = \lambda(t) + \lambda_E(t), \tag{3.3}$$

where $\lambda_E(t)$ is the expected mortality hazard for the general cancer-free population and $\lambda(t)$ is the excess hazard due to the cancer. Because a cohort of cancer-free individuals is difficult to obtain, life tables representing the survival of the general population are used to estimate expected survival. The underlying assumption is that cancer deaths are a negligible proportion of all deaths [13].

Relative survival is usually estimated by using the actuarial method and dividing the time after diagnosis into annual or monthly intervals. The expected survival can be obtained from a national life table and is usually calculated by matching for age, sex, year of diagnosis, and so forth. The main advantage of using relative survival is that the information on the cause of death is not required, circumventing problems with the inaccuracy or non-availability of death certificates.

Cancer incidence, survival and mortality are essential population-based indicators for public health and cancer control. These three measures are distinctive, but interconncected [8]. Confusion and misunderstanding still surround the estimation and interpretation of these three quantities. The relationship between the three measures can be described as a multistate model that includes transition from cancer-free state and death, including a possible intermediate status of cancer. Ellis et al. [8] described the concept that underlying the three measures illustrates the syngery among them.

Let S be the measure of survival, C be the number of new cancer cases, and D be the number of cancer patients dying from any cause in 5 years after diagnosis. Under the assumptions that all cancer patients only die from cancer of diagnosis with minimum follow-up of 5 years and the risk of dying from cancer is constant with 5 years, the 5-year survival rate can be calculated as $S = 1 - D / C$.

3.2 Statistical Methods for Population-Based Cancer Data

3.2.1 The Spatial Pattern of Cancer Incidence and Mortality

Spatial analysis of cancer incidence and mortality rates are important for the understanding of spatial and temporal distribution patterns and for the identification of underlying risk factors. The spatial heterogeneity across different regions may be due to population composition, age structure, and other socioeconomic factors. However, it is difficult to display and identify geospatial patterns and their associations with demographic, environmental. and other factors due to the multidimensionality of the complex data structure. First, the basic geospatial data are two-dimensional and including the temporal trend will add another dimension. In addition, the demographic, environmental, and other factors may be intercorrelated, adding the complexities of their associations with the outcome variable of interest. Linked micromap (LM) plots visually link geographic and statistical data and have been shown to be useful for both data exploration and presentation of georeferenced cancer statistics [14–17]. The LM allows users to view multiple variables interactively and compare statistics across regions, e.g., states, counties, registries, hospitals, and across time.

Carr et al. [15] reviewed the main features and use of the LM plots. The LM plots include at least three parallel sequences of panels that are linked by position. The three basic sequencies consist of micromaps, linking legends, and commonly used visual plots, e.g., times series plots for cancer trends. More sequences of panels can be included as long as the three basic panels exist. Within the panels of micromaps, distinct colors are used within perceptual groups of geographic units to link each region's name with its statistical graphic elements and map location. By sorting the geographic units in different ways, different patterns and trends of statistics can be revealed in the maps and the association between them. Because the LM plots are flexible and visually informative, they can be used for both exploratory data analysis and communication and presentation of cancer geospatial pattern. The state is often the preferred geographic unit for analysis and display of U.S. data. For data collected routinely across the entire U.S., state populations are large enough to show stable patterns for many types of cancer statistics while still protecting the privacy of cancer patients.

The LM plot has been implemented in R packages `micromapST` [18] and `micromap` [19] to display various cancer statistics for the 50 U.S. states plus the District of Columbia (DC). The entire plot fits on a single page in portrait orientation to support rapid visual queries. Each column in the design may address a different topic and the information displayed for each topic may consist of one or more statistical variables, a map, or a state name label. The graphic elements (glyphs) for each state/topic (row/column) combination may represent a single statistical value, e.g., by a dot or horizontal bar, with or without an uncertainty measure. Two values per state may be represented by an arrow indicating the change in values, e.g., between two timepoints, or by a scatter plot of the paired data. The distribution of substate values, e.g., for counties within each state, may be compared across states by means of box plots. Multiple pairs of state values can be shown as line graphs or scatter plots. The line graphs may represent, for example, a time series, a cumulative distribution, or a Q-Q plot of each state distribution relative to the national distribution. Categorical data can be represented as stacked bars. The user can choose the row sort order, column order, and the type of glyph used for each panel without having to be concerned about the sizing or spacing of the plot components required to create a publication-quality graphical display. The final layout may be saved in various popular image file formats.

3.2.2 Trends of Cancer Incidence and Mortality Rates

The most frequently asked question in the analysis of cancer statistics is whether the cancer trends are changing. Various methods have been used, but these methods have both merits and disadvantages. For example, both linear regression and polynomial regression have been used to depicit the trends of cancer incidence and mortality rates. A polynomial fit to the rate data has a continuously changing slope, which makes the interpretation difficult. In addition, the polynomial fits tend to have wider variability at the ends of the data series. A linear regression can be used to fit the logarithm of age-adjusted rates within a pre-specified interval. The resulting slope estimate can be interpreted by the annual percentage change (APC) of rate during the interval. However, the choice of the intervals is somewhat arbitrary rather than determined by the data, and the incidence and mortality rates for many cancer types indeed present a nonlinear trends.

To address the challenges of modeling cancer trends, Kim et al. [20] considered a piecewise linear model, where the linear segments join at the change points. They proposed a sequential testing procedure to select the number of segments and estimate the model parameters. For modeling the trends of incidence and mortality rates over time, the joinpoint model is specified as

$$y = \beta_0 + \beta_1 x + \sum_{k=1}^{K} \delta_k (x - \tau_k)^+ + \varepsilon, \tag{3.4}$$

where y is usually the logarithm of incidence or mortality rate; x is the time variable, e.g., calendar year; $z+ = \max(0, z)$; τ are the unknown locations of change points where segment mean functions change; and the number of change points, K, is assumed to be unknown. Let $\tau_0 = 0$ and $\tau_{K+1} = x_{max}$ be the minimum and maximum values of time variable x. Because the response is continuous at the change points τ_k, the change points are also called joinpoints and the model is called the joinpoint regression model.

The least-squares method can be used to fit the model for when the number and location of the joinpoints are known. To estimate the locations of k unknown joinpoints, $\tau_1, \cdots, \tau_K$, the grid search method [21] is used to find the joinpoints with the best least-square fit. The joinpoint estimates from the grid search method can only occur at the pre-determined grid, e.g., annual grid. A more accurate estimation method may allow the joinpoints to occur at any time during the observation period [22, 23]. The estimates of the regression coefficients are then obtained based on the estimated joinpoints. The residual sum of squares is obtained for a series of models with $K = 0, ..., K_{max}$ joinpoints, where K_{max} is the maximum number of joinpoints. Kim et al. [20] proposed a sequential testing procedure to determine the appropriate number of joinpoints. Because the procedure is based on multiple testings, the significance level of each test is adjusted to maintain the overall error rate of overfitting the model. Once the number of joinpoints is determined, asymptotic inference on regression parameters, including slope parameters and joinpoint locations, is performed. The p-values and confidence intervals (CIs) for the regression slopes are based on asymptotic normality. The joinpoint model has been implemented in the Joinpoint software, which can be downloaded from http://surveillance.cancer.gov/joinpoint/.

For the joinpoint model (3.4), the regression slope for segment $[\tau_{k-1}, \tau_k]$ is

$$\beta_k = \beta_1 + \sum_{j=1}^{k-1} \delta_j,$$

for $k = 1, ..., K + 1$. If the response variable y is the logarithm of the incidence or mortality rates and the time variable x is the calendar year, then the exponential of the regression coefficient $\exp(\beta_k)$ can be interpreted as the APC of incidence or mortality rates, i.e., $APC_k = \exp(\beta_k), k = 1, ..., K$. A summary measure called average annual percentage change (AAPC) can be calculated as the weighted geometric mean of the APC over a fixed pre-specified segment [24]. The AAPC measure can be used to compare recent trends of two or more series in the same time interval. The Annual Report to the Nation on the Status of Cancer, an annual publication summarizing trends in cancer rates, started reporting 5-year AAPCs in 2009 [25].

3.2.3 Cancer Survival Analysis and Predictions

Although the statistical methods are developed for cause-specific survival data where the responses are OS or cause-specific survival rate, various statistical methods have been adapted to the relative survival for population-based cancer survival data. The models may be classified into two groups: regression relative survival without cure and relative survival models with cure. Regression relative survival models are used to estimate the effect of covariates on survival and to predict survival in future calendar years. Cure survival models are used to estimate the proportion of subjects who are cured statistically and who have similar survival to the general cancer-free population. Most relative survival regression methods model the excess hazard $\lambda(t)$ of a cancer diagnosis [26, 27], which is defined in Eq. (3.3). For grouped survival data, Hakulinen and Tekanen [26] proposed using the binomial regression model with a complementary log-log link. Methods to estimate relative survival using individual data and the full likelihood approach have been developed by Dickman et al. [27] and Esteve et al. [28]. Recently, Nelson et al. [29] and Royston and Parmar [30] proposed flexible parametric models for relative survival data by fitting restricted cubic splines on the log cumulative excess hazard scale. The main advantages of these models are the ability to model time on a continuous scale and the possibility to incorporate time-varying covariates. Other methods have been recently developed to model relative survival with time-dependent effects [31–33].

Advances in early diagnosis and treatment often impact the survival of patients at a specific timepoint and then level off after those advances have been fully incorporated on a population level. Therefore, modeling survival trends and projecting up-to-date survival in the presence of a change point may facilitate understanding of the relationship between medical improvements and the survival experience for the patient population at large. Joinpoint models have recently been extended to model the progress of and trends in cancer survival rates [23]. The survival joinpoint models fit the piecewise linear regression model to the additive hazard of relative survival. Let $\lambda(t \mid x)$ be the hazard function at t years after cancer diagnosis for a subject who is diagnosed with cancer in calendar year x. The joinpoint survival model assumes that

$$\lambda(t \mid x) = \lambda_0(t)\exp\left\{\beta x + \sum_{k=1}^{K}\delta_k(x-\tau_k)^+\right\},$$

where x is the calendar year of cancer diagnosis, $(\tau_1,...,\tau_K)$ are the location of the joinpoints, $\lambda_0(t)$ is the baseline hazard, and $\beta, \delta_1,...,\delta_k$ are the parameters. This formulation is similar to the joinpoint regression models for incidence and mortality rates, but the response is survival after cancer diagnosis. The joinpoint survival model has been implemented in R package JPSurv (https://analysistools.cancer.gov/jpsurv/).

Due to improvement in cancer treatments and dissemination of early diagnosis techniques, there has been considerable progress against cancer. If diagnosed early and treated successfully, a proportion of patients may be cured for many types of cancer. The cure fraction is defined as the proportion of patients who are cured of disease and become long-term survivors. Failing to account for the cured patients may lead to incorrect inferences. Moreover, cure fraction itself is a useful measure of cancer control to researchers and policy makers. Note that the biological cure of cancer is usually achieved by eradicating cancer in the human body and cannot only be verified by long-term follow-up and immunohistochemical tests. By using the relative survival from the population-based cancer registry, the cure fraction can be interpreted as the proportion of patients whose survival becomes the same as that for the cancer-free population.

The mixture cure model was widely used to model the cancer net survival function $S(t)$ using population-based cancer survival data. Earlier work includes Boag [34], Berkson and Gage [35], and Cutler et al. [36]. Recently, Zhang and Peng [37] considered accelerated a hazards mixture cure model for population-based cancer survival data, Lambert et al. [38] discussed the application of non-mixture cure models, and Lambert et al. [39] developed a finite mixture cure model for population-based cancer survival data. There have been various applications of the mixture cure model for the projection of cancer rates and prevalences. De Angelis et al. [40] analyzed the survival of Finish colon cancer patients by adjusting for background mortality. The survival function for a mixture cure model is specified as

$$S(t \mid x) = c(x) + (1-c(x))S_u(t \mid x), \qquad (3.5)$$

where x is the vector of covariates, $c(x)$ is the cure fraction, and $S_u(t \mid x)$ is the survival function for the uncured patients (latent distribution). Let $f(t \mid x)$ and $\lambda(t \mid x)$ denote the density and hazard functions for the overall population, respectively. A logistic model is often used to model the cure fraction:

$$c(x) = \frac{\exp(\alpha' x)}{1 + \exp(\alpha' x)}, \qquad (3.6)$$

where $\alpha = (\alpha_1, ..., \alpha_{p_\alpha})$ is the vector of coefficients. The latent distribution $S_u(t)$ could be parametric or nonparametric (piecewise constant) [41, 42]. For example, for the Weibull latent survival model,

$$S_u(t \mid x) = \exp\left\{-\exp\left(\frac{\log t - \mu(x)}{\sigma}\right)\right\}.$$

Usually, we assume that the location parameter is related to covariates as

$$\mu(x) = \beta' x, \qquad (3.7)$$

where $\beta = (\beta_1, ..., \beta_{p_\beta})$ is the vector of regression coefficients. Note that the covariates used in $c(x)$ and $\mu(x)$ may not be identical. Hence, the analysts should pick the appropriate variables to be used in each component. The mixture cure model has been implemented in NCI-sponsored software CanSurv (https://surveillance.cancer.gov/cansurv/) [43].

3.3 Applications to Small Cell Lung Cancer

SCLC, sometimes called oat cell cancer, accounts for about 10% to 15% of lung cancers. SCLC is usually asymptomatic, which means it does not cause symptoms in early stages. Once symptoms do appear, it often is during late stages or the cancer has metastasized. SCLC is usually broken down into two stages, i.e., limited or extensive stages. In the limited stage, the cancer is confined to one side of your chest. The lymph nodes might also be affected. In the extensive stage, the cancer has spread to the other side of your chest, affecting the other lung. In extensive stages, the cancer has also invaded the lymph nodes as well as other parts of the body. If SCLC is detected in its early stages, the chances of making a recovery are much higher. However, SCLC is a very aggressive type of cancer and the survival rate is rather low in genearl. In this chapter, we present the cancer statistics, including the incidence, mortality, and survival, based on the population-based cancer registries in the Surveillance Epidemiology and End Results (SEER) Program [44].

We also analyze the IMpower 133 clinical trial that evaluates the efficacy of atezolizumab plus chemotherapy for treating first-line extensive-stage SCLC [45]. We intend to estimate the long-term survival for extensive-stage SCLC patients treated with atezolizumab. Because there is limited follow-up time for the complete ascertainment of OS status in the IMpower trial, the estimation of long-term survival relies on the modeling and extrapolation of survival curves in the clinical trials. We discuss the option of using RWE from the population-based cancer survival data to inform the extrapolation of long-term survival.

3.3.1 Spatial Patterns and Trends of SCLC Incidence and Mortality

We examine the spatial patterns and trends of SCLC incidence and IBM rates in the United States from 2001 to 2015. The incidence and mortality rates are extracted from the SEER*Stat software (http://seerstat.cancer.gov/seerstat/). First, we show the spatial pattern of distant stage SCLC incidence rates in the United States. Then we examine the trends of age-adjusted incidence rates and IBM rates for the entire United Staets using the joinpoint model. Figure 3.1 shows the LM of the SCLC incidence rate in distant stages by the 51 states including DC. Horizontally, the 51 regions are grouped into three blocks. Two large blocks at the top and bottom show the 25 states with high and low SCLC rates, respectively. A small block with one panel contains a single state with the median SCLC incidence rates. Each of the large blocks is further divided into panels of five states each.

The micromap has four columns. The leftmost column contains a series of small maps, one for each panel of five states. The U.S. state map is a modification of Monmonier's visibility map [46] with highly generalized boundaries and enlarged areas of extremely small states. Thus state shapes on the small maps are still recognizable and large enough that their color fills are readily identified. Each map is followed by a list of state names with a rectangle indicating the color of that state on the map for that panel in the second column. From the first two columns, we see that the states in the central U.S. region have the highest SCLC incidence rates. According to the American Cancer Society, smoking is by far the leading risk factor for lung cancer. About 80% of all lung cancer deaths are thought to result from smoking, and this number is probably even higher for SCLC. It is very rare for someone who has never smoked to have SCLC. The states with the highest SCLC rates overlap highly with the states with the highest cigarette smoking rates among adults (https://www.cdc.gov/statesystem/cigaretteuseadult.html). Particularly, we see that the five states with the highest SCLC rates, i.e., Kentucy, West Virginia, Indiana, Missouri, and Tennessee, are also among the list with the highest smoking rates. This clearly shows the correlation between smoking and SCLC. From the cancer prevention perspective, it is imperative to reduce the smoking rate to successfully decrease the SCLC incidence. This also indicates that the central region imposes the highest SCLC cancer burden.

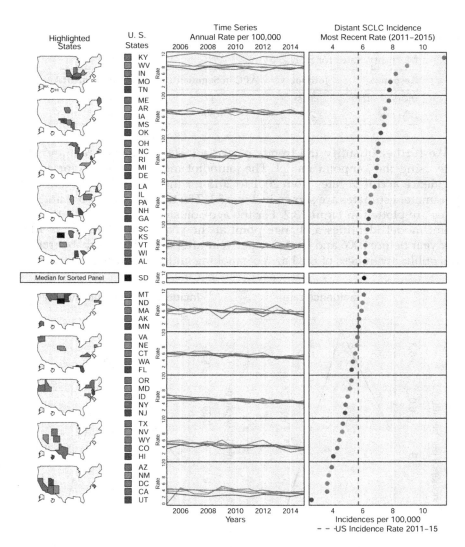

FIGURE 3.1
Age-adjusted distant stage SCLC incidence rates.

The third column shows the trends of age-adjusted SCLC rates from 2001 to 2015. We see that SCLC incidence rates decreased slightly over the 15-year period. This indicates that SCLC remains a big cancer burden in spite of the steady decrease. The last column shows that the latest SCLC incidence rates for the 51 states from 2011 to 2015. Kentucky has the highest SCLC rate at 12 cases per 100,000 per year. The median SCLC rate for the entire United States is about 6.2 cases per 100,000.

TABLE 3.1

Joinpoint Model Fit for the Incidence Rate and Incidence-Based Mortality Rates for SCLC

Response	Joinpoint	APC in Segment 1	APC in Segment 2
Incidence rate	2006	1.17	−1.91
IBM rate	2009	0.80	−2.10

We further quantify the trends of age-adjusted incidence rate and IBM rate using the joinpoint model. The joinpoint model is used to for annual incidence and IBM rates from 2001 to 2015 for the entire United States. The parameter estimates are shown in Table 3.1. The trends of incidence and IBM rates are plotted in Figure 3.2. For the age-adjusted incidence rate, the joinpoint model identifies a change point at the year 2006. The APC is 1.17% per year before 2006 and is −1.91% per year after 2006. This probably reflects the public awareness of the harm of smoking and the increasing availability

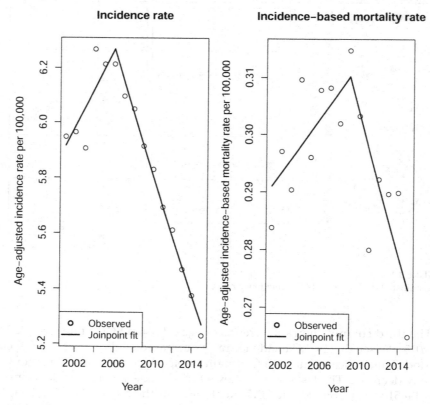

FIGURE 3.2

Fit of joinpoint models for the SCLC incidence and IBM rates.

of smoking cessation resources. The trends of the IBM rate follow a similar pattern and has a change point at the year 2009, which is 3 years behind the change point in 2006 for incidence rate.

3.3.2 Trends of SCLC Survival Using Population-Based Registry Data

The trends of SCLC survival is a measure of cancer treatment progress over time. We use the survival data for extensive-stage SCLC patients diagnosed from 2000 to 2015 for the analysis. The maximum follow-up time is 15 years. A survival joinpoint model is used to estimate the trends. Based on the Bayesian information criterion, the survival joinpoint model does not identify a change point. The k-year survival rates for the SCLC patients, $k = 0.5, 1, 5$, are shown in Figure 3.3. Over the 15-year period, we see slight improvement in survival rate. The half-year survival rates remain around 50%, and the 5-year survival rates are all below 5%. For the patients diagnosed in 2015, the predicted 5-year survival rate is only 3.2%. The APC of the survival rate is only 0.17% with a standard error of 0.03%. Although highly statistically significant because of the large number of patients, the slight improvement of 0.17% indicates that there is little progress in cancer treatment for SCLC and it remains a significant unmet patients' need.

Because that diagnosis year is not strongly associated with the improvement of survival, we pool all the survival data for patients diagnosed from 2000 to 2015 and fit parametric survival models. We consider the Weibull

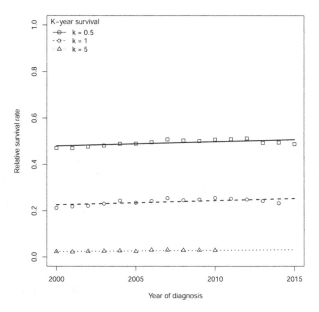

FIGURE 3.3
Trends of k-year survival for the SCLC patients.

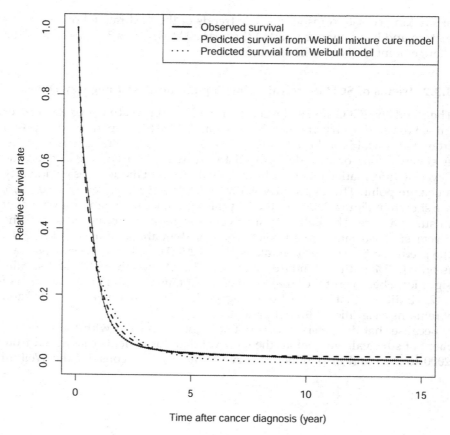

FIGURE 3.4
Fit of parametric survival models for the SCLC survival.

model with and without cure. The fit of the parametric survival models in shown in Figure 3.4. The solid line is the observed survival curve and the dashed and dotted lines are the predicted survival rates from the Weibull mixture cure model and the Weibull model, respectively. With the mixture cure model, the estimate of cure fraction is only 2%. We can see that the two Weibull models, i.e, with and without cure, provide similar fit to the observed survival data. The median survivial time is only 4.9 months. This indicates that extensive-stage SCLC remains uncurable based on the current available therapy until the year 2015.

3.3.3 Extrapolation of Long-Term Survival for an SCLC Clinical Trial

IMPower 133 is a double-blind, placebo-controlled, phase 3 trial to evaluate atezolizumab plus carboplatin (CP) and etoposide (ET) in patients with extensive-stage SCLC who had not previously received treatment [45]. Patients are randomly assigned in a 1:1 ratio to receive CP and ET with either atezolizumab or placebo for four 21-day cycles (induction phase), followed by a maintenance phase during which they receive either atezolizumab or placebo (according to the previous random assignment) until they had unacceptable toxic effects, disease progression according to Response Evaluation Criteria in Solid Tumors version 1.1, or no additional clinical benefit. The two primary endpoints are investigator-assessed PFS and OS in the intention-to-treat population. A total of 201 patients are randomly assigned to the atezolizumab group, and 202 patients to the placebo group. At a median follow-up of 13.9 months, the median OS is 12.3 months in the atezolizumab group and 10.3 months in the placebo group. The hazard ratio of death is 0.70 with 95% CI (0.54, 0.91) and p-value = 0.007. Based on the published OS curves [45], the OS data are reconstructed using the algorithm described by Guyot et al. [47]. The Kaplan-Meier curves of the placebo and atezolumab groups for the reconstructed IMPower 133 OS data are shown in Figure 3.5. We see that the Kaplan-Meier curves begin to diverge after month 5.

The clinical trial data may provide evidence for the efficacy of the innovative treatment during the study period, but it cannot provide the estimate of long-term cost-effectiveness of the treatment. Cost-effectiveness analysis is an important tool to compare the relative cost and effects of different health technologies and to provide a method of prioritizing the allocation of limited

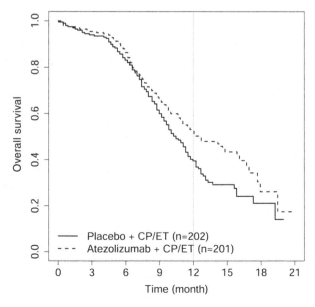

FIGURE 3.5
Kaplan-Meier curves of the reconstructed IMpower 133 overall survival data.

resources for more effective healthcare. The incremental cost-effectiveness ratio (ICER) is a commonly used measure of cost-effectiveness, where

$$\text{ICER} = \frac{E(C_{ID} - C_{SoC})}{E(B_{ID} - B_{SoC})}, \tag{3.8}$$

where C means cost and B means benefit, ID means innovative drug, and SoC means standard of care. In the setting of SCLC treatment, the ID is the atezolizmab + CP/ET and SoC is standard chemotherapy with CP/ET. The cost is usually expressed in the amount of money used, and benefit is measured as gained life years (LYs) or quality-adjusted life years (QALYs). For example, the Lys for comparing the benefit of survival is calculated as the area under the OS curves.

Survival analysis forms the basis of estimates of LY and QALY for health economics analysis and decision-making in reimbursement. Because the survival data from a clinical trial usually have limited duration, it is challenging to extrapolate to ensure that the long-term economic value of the cancer treatment is appropriately captured. For example, the follow-up time for the IMpower133 trial is about 20 months and the Kaplan-Meier estimate of survival is about 20% at month 20. Therefore, the long-term cost-effectiveness still requires extrapolation of survival. Because of limited follow-up time in clinical trials, reliable evidence to determine long-term cost-effectiveness is often absent at the time of submission for market authorization. Because the evidence is critically related to the pricing of cancer drugs and under intensive debate, it is crucial for decision makers to assess the true economic values of cancer treatment with rigorous and robust methods.

If we rely only on the information from clinical trials, one may fit the statistical models to the limited survival data from clinical trial and extrapolate the survival beyond the follow-up time. Figure 3.6 shows the survival extrapolation based on the Weibull model for the clinical trial survival data. The fit of the Weibull model is good during the trial period of less than 22 months. The survival curves for both arms are close to 0 at month 36. Even for such a short extrapolation, people may question the reliability of the extrapolation because very few people survive beyond month 24. The RWD from the population-based cancer registry may provide valuable information about the long-term survival rate. We are able to extract the long-term survival data from the SEER 13 registries. The bottom dashed line in Figure 3.6 shows the observed OS data for patients with extensive-stage SCLC diagnosed from 2001 to 2015 in the SEER program. Because of little progress in treatment for SCLC as shown in Figure 3.3, we expect that mode of treatment is chemotherapy for the SEER data. Note that the observed survival from the SEER data is below the survival for the chemotherapy (Placebo + CP/ET) group. This is probably because of the patient difference or unmeasured difference between the clinical trial and real-world practice. However, we see the observed survival curve for the SEER data and the fitted survival

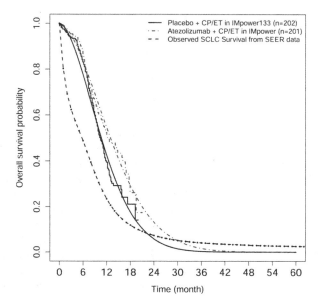

FIGURE 3.6
Comparison of the observed survival from SEER and survival curves based on the Weibull model for IMpower 133 trial.

curves from the chemotherapy arm in the IMpower133 trial cross at months 24. This may raise questions about the survival extrapolation based solely on the clinical trials. If the same treatment mode is used in the clinical trial chemotherapy group and the SEER data, we expect the survival surves will be more or less proportional. Therefore, we expect that the long-term survival rate for the placebo arm in the IMPower 133 clinical trial will be slightly above the observed long-term SCLC survival from SEER data. Let λ_O, λ_P and λ_A denote the hazard rate for the observed SCLC survival from SEER data as the hazard rates for the placebo and atezolizumab groups in the IMPower 133 trial, respectively. Let $\hat{\lambda}_P(t)$ and $\hat{\lambda}_A(t)$ be the estimated hazard functions and let $\hat{\delta}$ be the hazard ratio estimate from the Weibull model for the IMpower 133 trial. We assume that $\lambda_P(t) = \lambda_O(t)$ and $\lambda_A(t) = \delta\lambda_P(t)$, for $t > 18$ months. This implies that the placebo group has the same hazard rate as the patients from the SEER data. The hazard ratio δ represents the effect of atezolizumab versus the placebo group in the IMPower 133 trial, which can be estimated from the trial data. By substituting the long-term hazard rate from the SEER data to the hazard rate for the placebo group, we get

$$\lambda_P(t) = \begin{cases} \hat{\lambda}_P(t) & t \leq 18 \\ \lambda_O(t) & t > 18 \end{cases}$$

(3.9)

and

$$\lambda_A(t) = \begin{cases} \hat{\lambda}_A(t) & t \le 18 \\ \delta\lambda_O(t) & t > 18 \end{cases} \tag{3.10}$$

By concatenating the short-term survival data from the clinical trial and the long-term survival data from the population-based cancer registry, the OS for the placebo and atezolizumab groups from the IMpower 133 trials are extrapolated to 5 years. The extrapolation of the OS rates are shown in Figure 3.7. The black solid line is the adjusted OS curves for the placebo + CP/ET group and the blue dash line is the adjusted survival curve for the Atezolizumab + CP/ET, after incoporating the long-term survival data from the population-based cancer registry. Now there is no crossover in survival curves, which is more compatible to the proportional hazards assumption. Guyot et al. [48] considered various choices for the relationship between the hazard functions of clinical trial data and external data. However, they emphasized that using external data for extrapolation requires subjective

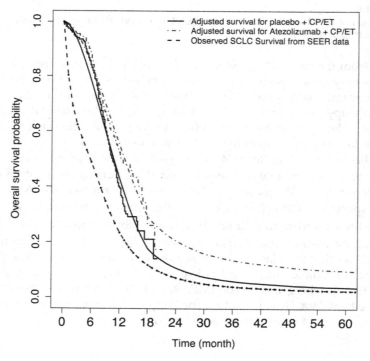

FIGURE 3.7
Extrapolation of overall survival for the placebo and atezolizumab groups by incorporating long-term survival data from the population-based cancer registry.

judgment about the relevance and applicability of the data. The survival exp-trapolation may be sensitive to the assumption, therefore, the assumptions must be open to examination, debate, and sensitivity analysis.

3.4 Summary

In this chapter, we introduced several commonly used cancer statistics for measuring the cancer burden and the progress against cancer. The incidence, mortality, and survival derived from the population-based cancer registry data are representative for the general population and provide the RWE of the impact of cancer. We described statistical methods, e.g., the micro-linked map and the joinpoint model, for the analysis and presentation of cancer statistics.

We also presented a simple example to show that the RWD from the population-based cancer registry may supplement the information from clinical trials to inform the long-term survival extrapolation for cancer patients. By combining the data from clinical trials and population-based cancer registries, we may provide a more reasonable estimate of long-term survival. This may be used as a sensitivity analysis for the estimate of ICER in cost-effectiveness analysis.

Bibliography

1. DeVita, V.T. 2004. The 'war on cancer' and its impact. *Nature Clinical Practice Oncology*, 1(2), 55–55, December.
2. Bouchardy, C., Rapiti, E., and Benhamou, S. 2014. Cancer registries can provide evidence-based data to improve quality of care and prevent cancer deaths. *eCancer Medical Science*, 8, 413.
3. U.S. FDA. 2019. *Submitting Documents using Real-World Data and Real-World Evidence to FDA for Drugs and Biologics*. U.S. Department of Health and Human Services, FDA, Silver Spring, MD 20993.
4. Stower, H. 2019. The promise of real-world data. *Nature Medicine*, Online ahead of print. doi: 10.1038/d41591-019-00010-z
5. Skovlund, E., Leufkens, H.G.M., and Smyth, J.F. 2018. The use of real-world data in cancer drug development. *European Journal of Cancer*, 101, 69–76.
6. Booth, C.M., Karim, S., and Mackillop, W.J. 2019. Real-world data: towards achieving the achievable in cancer care. *Nature Reviews Clinical Oncology*, 16(5), 312–325.
7. Parkin, D.M. 2006. The evolution of the population-based cancer registry. *Nature Reviews Cancer*, 6(8), 603–612.
8. Ellis, L., Woods, L.M., Estève, J., Eloranta, S., Coleman, M.P., and Rachet, B. 2014. Cancer incidence, survival and mortality: Explaining the concepts. *International Journal of Cancer*, 135(8), 1774–1782.

9. Anderson, R.N. and Rosenberg, H. M. 1998. Age standardization of death rates: implementation of the year 2000 standard. *National Vital Statistics Reports*, 47(3), 1–16.

10. Chu, K. C., Miller, B.A., Feuer, E.J., and Hankey, B.F. 1994. A method for partitioning cancer mortality trends by factors associated with diagnosis: an application to female breast cancer. *Journal of Clinical Epidemiology*, 47(12), 1451–1461.

11. Chen, H.S., Mariotto, A.B., Zhu, L., Kim, H.J., Cho, H., and Feuer, E.J. 2014. Developments and challenges in statistical methods in cancer surveillance. *Statistics and Its Interface*, 7(1), 135–151.

12. Begg, C.B. and Schrag, D. 2002. Attribution of deaths following cancer treatment. *Journal of the National Cancer Institute*, 94(14), 1044–1045.

13. Ederer, F. 1961. The relative survival rate: a statistical methodology. *NCI Monograph*, 6, 101–121.

14. Carr, D.B. and Pierson, S.M. 1996. Emphasizing statistical summaries and showing spatial context with micromaps. *Statistical Computing and Graphics Newsletter*, 7(3), 16–23.

15. Carr, D.B., Olsen, A.R., Courbois, J.P., Pierson, S.M., and Carr, D.A. 1998. Linked micromap plots: named and described. *Statistical Computing and Graphics Newsletter*, 9(1), 24–32.

16. Carr, D.B., Wallin, J.F., and Carr, D.A. 2000. Two new templates for epidemiology applications: linked micromap plots and conditioned choropleth maps. *Statistics in Medicine*, 19(17–18), 2521–2538.

17. Carr, D.B. and Pickle, L.W. 2010. *Visualizing Data Patterns with Micromaps*. London: Chapman and Hall.

18. Carr, Jr, D.B., Pearson, J.B., and Pickle, L.W. 2013. Micromapst: state linked micromap plots. *R Package Version*, 1, 02.

19. Payton, Q.C., McManus, M.G., Weber, M.H., Olsen, A.R., and Kincaid, T.M. 2015. Micromap: a package for linked micromaps. *Journal of Statistical Software*, 63(2).

20. Kim, H.-J., Fay, M.P., Feuer, E.J., and Midthune, D.N. 2000. Permutation tests for joinpoint regression with applications to cancer rates. *Statistics in Medicine*, 19(3), 335–351.

21. Lerman, P.M. 1980. Fitting segmented regression models by grid search. *Applied Statistics*, 29(1), 77–84.

22. Hudson, D.J. 1966. Fitting segmented curves whose join points have to be estimated. *Journal of the American Statistical Association*, 61(316), 1097–1129.

23. Yu, B., Barrett, M.J., Kim, H.-J., and Feuer, E.J. 2007. Estimating joinpoints in continuous time scale for multiple change-point models. *Computational Statistics and Data Analysis*, 51(5), 2420–2427.

24. Clegg, L.X., Hankey, B.F., Tiwari, R., Feuer, E.J., and Edwards, B.K. 2009. Estimating average annual per cent change in trend analysis. *Statistics in Medicine*, 28(29), 3670–3682.

25. Cronin, K.A. Lake, A.J., Scott, S., Sherman, R.L., Noone, A.M., Howlader, N.S., Henley, J., Anderson, R.N., Firth, A.U., Ma, J, Kohler, B.A., and Jemal, A. 2018. Annual report to the nation on the status of cancer. Part I: national cancer statistics. *Cancer*, 124(13), 2785–2800.

26. Hakulinen T. and Tenkanen, L. 1987. Regression analysis of relative survival rates. *Applied Statistics*, 36, 309–317.

27. Dickman, P.W., Sloggett, A., Hills, M., and Hakulinen, T. 2004. Regression models for relative survival. *Statistics in Medicine*, 23(1), 51–64.
28. Estve, J., Benhamou, E., Croasdale, M., and Raymond, L. 1990. Relative survival and the estimation of net survival: Elements for further discussion. *Statistics in Medicine*, 9(5), 529–538.
29. Nelson, C.P., Lambert, P.C., Squire, I.B., and Jones, D.R. 2007. Flexible parametric models for relative survival, with application in coronary heart disease. *Statistics in Medicine*, 26(30), 5486–5498.
30. Royston, P. and Parmar, M.K.B. 2002. Flexible parametric proportional-hazards and proportional-odds models for censored survival data, with application to prognostic modelling and estimation of treatment effects. *Statistics in Medicine*, 21(15), 2175–2197.
31. Giorgi, R., Payan, J., and Gouvernet, J. 2005. RSURV: a function to perform relative survival analysis with S-plus or R. *Computer Methods and Programs in Biomedicine*, 78(2), 175–178.
32. Pohar, M. and Stare, J. 2006. Relative survival analysis in R. *Computer Methods and Programs in Biomedicine*, 81(3), 272–278.
33. Pohar, M. and Stare, J. 2007. Making relative survival analysis relatively easy. *Computers in Biology and Medicine*, 37(12), 1741–1749.
34. Boag, J.W. 1949. Maximum likelihood estimates of the proportion of patients cured by cancer therapy. *Journal of the Royal Statistical Society, Series B*, 11, 15–44.
35. Berkson, J. and Gage, R.P. 1952. Survival curve for cancer patients following treatment. *Journal of the American Statistical Association*, 47, 501–515.
36. Cutler, S.J., Axtell, L.M., and Schottenfeld, D. 1969. Adjustment of long-term survival rates for deaths due to intercurrent disease. *Journal of Chronic Diseases*, 22(6–7), 485–491.
37. Zhang, J. and Peng, Y. 2009. Accelerated hazards mixture cure model. *Lifetime Data Analysis*, 15(4), 455–467.
38. Lambert, P.C., Thompson, J.R., Weston, C.L., and Dickman, P.W. 2007. Estimating and modeling the cure fraction in population-based cancer survival analysis. *Biostatistics*, 8(3), 576–594.
39. Lambert, P.C., Dickman, P.W., Nelson, C.P., and Royston, P. 2010. Estimating the crude probability of death due to cancer and other causes using relative survival models. *Statistics in Medicine*, 29(7–8), 885–895.
40. De Angelis, R., Capocaccia, R., Hakulinen, T., Soderman, B., and Verdecchia, A. 1999. Mixture models for cancer survival analysis: application to population-based data with covariates. *Statistics in Medicine*, 18(4), 441–454.
41. Peng, Y. and Dear, K.B. 2000. A nonparametric mixture model for cure rate estimation. *Biometrics*, 56(1), 237–243.
42. Zhang, J. and Peng, Y. 2007. A new estimation method for the semiparametric accelerated failure time mixture cure model. *Statistics in Medicine*, 26(16), 3157–3171.
43. Yu, B., Tiwari, R.C., Cronin, K.A., McDonald, C., and Feuer, E.J. 2005. CanSurv: a windows program for population-based cancer survival analysis. *Computer Methods and Programs in Biomedicine*, 80(3), 195–203.
44. Gloeckler Ries, L.A. 2003. Cancer survival and incidence from the surveillance, epidemiology, and end results (SEER) program. *The Oncologist*, 8(6), 541–552.
45. Horn, L., Mansfield, A.S., Szczesna, A., Havel, L., Krzakowski, M., Hochmair, M.J., Huemer, F., Losonczy, G., Johnson, M.L., Nishio, M., Reck, M., Mok, T.,

Lam, S., Shames, D.S., Liu, J., Ding, B., Lopez-Chavez, A., Kabbinavar, F., Lin, W., Sandler, A., and Liu, S.V. 2018. First-line atezolizumab plus chemotherapy in extensive-stage small-cell lung cancer. *New England Journal of Medicine*, 379(23), 2220–2229.

46. Monmonier, M. 1988. Geographical representations in statistical graphics: a conceptual framework. *Proceedings of the Section on Statistical Graphics*, 1–10.

47. Guyot, P., Ades, A. E., Ouwens, M.J.N.M., and Welton, N.J. 2012. Enhanced secondary analysis of survival data: reconstructing the data from published Kaplan-Meier survival curves. *BMC Medical Research Methodology*, 12(1), 9.

48. Guyot, P., Ades, A.E., Beasley, M., Lueza, B., Pignon, J.-P., and Welton, N.J. 2017. Extrapolation of survival curves from cancer trials using external information. *Medical Decision Making*, 37(4), 353–366.

4

External Control Using RWE and Historical Data in Clinical Development

Qing Li, Guang Chen, Jianchang Lin, Andy Chi, Simon Davies

4.1 Introduction of Using RWE and Historical Data in Clinical Development

In December 2016, the 21st Century Cures Act was signed into law (Food and Drug Administration [FDA] 2016). The act is designed to accelerate medical product development and to bring innovation faster to patients who have medical needs. In this document, Real-world data (RWD) and real-world evidence (RWE) were raised to support regulatory decision-making. In December 2018, the FDA released a new strategic framework to advance the use of RWE to support development of drugs and biologics (FDA 2018a). In 2019, the FDA also published a draft guidance on submitting documents using RWD and RWE to FDA (FDA 2019b). External control using RWE and historical data are playing an important role in the clinical development and drug evaluation.

This chapter presents an overview of how to adopt external control using RWD and historical control in clinical development. Randomized clinical trials are considered the gold standard for clinical development. However, recruiting a large number of subjects into a randomized clinical trial can be challenging, especially for orphan drug enrollment, certain subtype diseases, and rare diseases. Moreover, it is sometimes unethical or not feasible to conduct such a randomized clinical trial with a parallel control arm. When there are no approved drugs for a certain life-threating rare disease, randomizing patients into a placebo group may raise ethical concerns (FDA 2014b). Despite the challenges of conducting randomized clinical trials, there are also common limitations of traditional clinical research, including generalizability of clinical research findings and rapidly rising cost of both time and money. Due to the strict inclusion and exclusion criteria in clinical trials, patients in clinical trials are restricted and may not reflect the real clinical practice. Using RWD in clinical development can reflect the actual treatment effect in the real-world setting. Therefore, many researchers have become interested in integrating RWD with traditional clinical research in more diverse scenarios.

Borrowing RWE and historical control also can contribute to a more precise effect size estimation, endpoint selection, biomarker identification, and patient selection, thus helping to improve clinical trial recruitment and reduce sample size. In recent years, there have been drug approval cases using RWE or historical data as the control arm without adopting a standard parallel control arm in a clinical trial. These cases were primarily in oncology or rare disease settings. In this chapter, the use of external control in clinical development and approval will be demonstrated in two parts: (1) single-arm trials using external control for the new drug application (NDA)/biologic license application (BLA) and (2) comparison across trials with historical control for label expansion. At the end, we will also provide the important considerations when designing studies and analyzing data using external control in clinical development including study selection, comparability of the data, choice of propensity score model, baseline covariates selection and checking, sensitivity analysis and prospectively plan of study using external control.

4.2 Single-Arm Trial Using External Control for Initial Indication

Most of the time, randomized clinical trials are preferred as the basis of an NDA submission. There have been cases of trials that adopted single-arm designs that were successfully approved in FDA expedited programs for drugs and biologics treating serious conditions and fulfilling unmet medical need (FDA 2014a). However, it could be difficult to construct an objective reference level to compare with a single-arm study. In this situation, it would be helpful to employ an external control as a comparison arm instead of presenting just the single experimental arm. These external control arms could include historical clinical trials, natural history studies, patient registry data, and other types of RWD. In this section, we will exemplify three approved drugs that used a single-arm trial design with external control for an NDA. Each example with its unique features illustrates the challenges of using external control in clinical development. The Strensiq® case in Section 4.2.1 will demonstrate the contribution of an objective endpoint and dramatically higher treatment effect than commonly seen in randomized clinical trials to the successful drug approval. The Brineura® case in Section 4.2.2 will illustrate the challenges of comparability of endpoints between an active arm and historical control arm when an external control arm was used. The Bavencio® case in Section 4.2.3 will introduce the use of historical registry data to provide supportive evidence for a single-arm study.

4.2.1 Strensiq® for the Treatment of Patients with Perinatal, Infantile, and Juvenile Onset Hypophosphatasia (HPP)

HPP is a rare inherited genetic disorder that affects the development of bones and teeth. Since its discovery in 1936, no drug has been approved for the treatment of HPP. In October 2015, the FDA approved Strensiq® (asfotase alfa) for the treatment of patients with perinatal, infantile, and juvenile onset HPP (FDA 2015). It is the first approved drug for HPP disease in the United States. Strensiq® is an innovative enzyme replacement therapy (ERT) developed by Alexin Pharmaceuticals, Inc. This NDA received both rare pediatric disease priority review and breakthrough therapy designation.

The efficacy and safety evidence contained within the Strensiq® NDA submission was not based on a traditional randomized, controlled phase 3 trial. Instead, data came from four clinical trials comprised of patients with perinatal-, infantile-, and juvenile-onset HPP. Table 4.1 summarizes the relevant trial information. Table 4.1 shows that the ENB-002-08/ENB-003-08 and ENB-010-10 studies were single-arm studies. The objectives of these studies were to determine the efficacy (along with safety, long-term tolerability, and pharmacokinetics [PK]) of asfotase alfa in treating the skeletal manifestations of patients with perinatal/infantile-onset HPP. Of note, there were no concurrent control arms in these studies; they were single-arm studies due to the lack of standard of care for patients with HPP.

To determine the efficacy of asfotase alfa, a comparison group was needed to demonstrate the clinical benefits to patients. A natural history study (ENB-011-10) served as an external control group. To conduct a fair comparison, 48 patients were extracted from ENB-011-10 based on the similarities of the patient population to the asfotase alfa study patients, namely, patients with perinatal/infantile-onset HPP. The efficacy analyses were based on this integrated historical-controlled data set. Two patients from the overall 70-patient ENB-002-08/ENB-003-08 and ENB-010-10 pooled cohort did not qualify for the analysis due to failure to meet the entry/extraction criteria for natural history study ENB-011-10.

Table 4.2 shows that the demographic and baseline characteristics are balanced between the two arms for age and race, while the geographic region was imbalanced. However, this geographic region variable was not considered as critical as the other variables in terms of affecting treatment effects. By selecting the patients with similar demographic and baseline characteristics, the two arms were considered comparable.

The primary endpoint was time to death, from birth up to the point of last contact (i.e., overall survival [OS]), and the secondary endpoint was time to the start of invasive ventilator use or death (i.e., invasive ventilator-free survival). Both time-to-event endpoints were estimated using survival rates (i.e., the percentage of patients who did not experience the event of interest in either context), median survival time, hazard ratio, Kaplan-Meier curve, and log-rank test. In Table 4.3, the treatment arm using asfotase alfa showed

TABLE 4.1

Summary of the Relevant Study Information for Strensiq® Study

Type of study phase	Study Identifier	Objectives	Study Design and Type of Control	Test products; Regimen; Route	Number of patients	Patients Diagnosis	Duration of Treatment
Safety and efficacy; phase 2	ENB-002-08/ ENB-003-08	Efficacy, safety, PK	Multinational, multicenter, open-label, single-arm	Asfotase alfa: one 2 mg/kg infusion followed by 1 mg/kg/day SC injections 3 times per week with escalation up to 3mg/kg/day; SC injection	11	Perinatal/ infantile-onset HPP	24 weeks (ENB-002-08) with additional long-term extension up to 5 years (ENB-003-08)
Safety and efficacy; phase 2	ENB-010-10	Efficacy, safety, PK	Multinational, multicenter, open-label, single-arm	Asfotase alfa: 6 mg/kg/week administered as either 1 mg/kg 6 times per week or 2 mg/kg 3 times per week by SC injection; SC injection	59	Perinatal/ infantile-onset HPP	4 years
Natural history	ENB-011-10	Retrospective chart Review of patients with perinatal/ infantile-onset HPP	Observational, natural history, non-interventional	N/A	48	Perinatal/ infantile-onset HPP	N/A
Safety and efficacy; phase 2	ENB-006-09/ ENB-008-10	Efficacy, safety, PK	Multinational, multicenter, open-label, randomized, parallel-dose	Asfotase alfa: 2 or 3 mg/kg SC asfotase alfa 3 times per week (i.e., 6 or 9 mg/kg/week); SC injection	8	Juvenile-onset HPP	24 weeks (ENB-006-09) with additional long-term extension up to 3.5 years (ENB-008-10)
Natural history	ALX-HPP-502	Retrospective chart Review of patients with juvenile-onset HPP	Observational, natural history, non-interventional	N/A	32	Juvenile-onset HPP	N/A

TABLE 4.2

Demographic and Baseline Characteristics – ENB-002-08/ENB-003-08 and ENB-010-10 vs. ENB-011-10 (All Qualified Enrolled/Extracted)

	ENB-002-08/ENB-003-08 and ENB-010-10 Asfotase Alfa (N = 68)	ENB-011-10 Historical Control (N = 48)
Age at Symptom Onset (months)		
N	68	48
Mean (SD)	1.6 (1.69)	1.1 (1.67)
Median	1.0	0.03
Min, Max	0, 6	0, 6
Gender – n (%)		
Female	37 (54.4%)	22 (45.8%)
Male	31 (45.6%)	26 (54.2%)
Race – n (%)		
American Indian or Alaskan Native	0	1 (2.1%)
Asian	7 (10.3%)	2 (4.2%)
Black or African American	0	3 (6.3%)
Native Hawaiian or Other Pacific Islander	0	0
Other	2 (2.9%)	2 (4.2%)
White	54 (79.4%)	40 (83.3%)
Unknown	5 (7.4%)	0
Geographical Region – n (%)		
Europe	27 (39.7%)	8 (16.7%)
North America	35 (51.5%)	37 (77.1%)
Other	6 (8.8%)	3 (6.3%)

superior treatment effects in terms of all the OS measurements. The asfotase alfa treatment arm additionally had superior treatment effects for all the ventilator-free survival measurements, as seen in Table 4.4.

These primary and secondary endpoints are objective survival endpoints. The endpoints show direct clinical benefits to the survival of patients, which indicate the robust clinical evidence. The huge treatment effect also can be seen in all summary statistics, which is critical for successful Health Authority approval using an external control arm. Because the study design with an external control arm is not as rigid as a randomized clinical trial, the use of a historical control is considered by the FDA as a weaker level of evidence, as noted in the FDA statistical reviewer comments. The huge treatment effects also enable the conclusion to hold even if different sensitivity analyses were to be performed. The credibility of hypothesis testing with external control also is limited. All previously presented inferential statistics (e.g., *p*-values) within this example are considered supportive and not confirmatory, and no inferential statistics should be presented within the final product labeling.

TABLE 4.3

Overall Survival – ENB-002-08/ENB-003-08 and ENB-010-10 vs. ENB-011-10 (All Qualified Enrolled/Extracted)

	ENB-002-08/ENB-003-08 and ENB-010-10 Asfotase Alfa (N = 68)	ENB-011-10 Historical Control (N = 48)
Alive at Point of Last Contact – n (%)	62 (91.2%)	13 (27.1%)
Corresponding 95% CI [1]	(81.4%, 97.3%)	(15.3%, 41.9%)
Time to Death from Birth (in Days)		
N	68	48
Mean (SD)	1397.3(949.06)	1113.1 (1891.23)
Median	1353.0	270.5
Min, max	73, 3487*	1, 7211*
Hazard ratio (Asfotase Alfa/historical control)	0.089	
Corresponding 95% CI	(0.039, 0.202)	
Log-rank test *p*-value [2]	<0.0001	

4.2.2 Brineura® for a Specific Form of Batten Disease

Batten disease, which is also called neuronal ceroid lipofuscinoses (NCLs), is a family of rare, fatal, inherited disorders of the nervous system. It is estimated that 2–4 births per 100,000 in the United States are affected by Batten disease, which is considered as a rare disease. Batten disease was

TABLE 4.4

Invasive Ventilator-Free Survival – ENB-002-08/ENB-003-08 and ENB-010-10 versus ENB-011-10 (All Qualified Enrolled/Extracted)

	ENB-002-08/ENB-003-08 and ENB-010-10 Asfotase Alfa (N = 68)	ENB-011-10 Historical Control (N = 48)
Alive at Point of Last Contact – n (%)	45 (66.2%)	12 (25.0%)
Corresponding 95% CI [1]	(54.6%, 78.2%)	(13.6%, 39.6%)
Time to Death from Birth (in Days)		
N	68	48
Mean (SD)	1234.8 (989.95)	930.6 (1725.85)
Median	1078.0	236.0
Min, max	21, 3487*	1, 7211*
Hazard Ratio (Asfotase Alfa/historical control)	0.278	
Corresponding 95% CI	(0.162, 0.478)	
Log-rank test *p*-value [2]	<0.0001	

named after British pediatrician Frederick Batten, who first described the disease in 1903; however, there were no approved drugs until recently. In April 2017, the FDA approved Brineura® (cerliponase alfa), which was developed by BioMarin Pharmaceutical, Inc. as a treatment for a specific form of Batten disease (FDA 2017c). It is the first FDA-approved treatment to slow the loss of walking ability (ambulation) in symptomatic pediatric patients 3 years of age and older with late infantile neuronal ceroid lipofuscinosis type 2 (CLN2), also known as tripeptidyl peptidase-1 (TPP1) deficiency. The BLA of Brineura® received priority review and breakthrough therapy designation.

Similar to the Strensiq® application, the Brineura® BLA submission was not based on a traditional phase 3, randomized clinical trial. Instead, this application includes data from a phase 1/2, first-in-human, single-arm, open-label, dose-escalation (Study 201) trial and a treatment extension study (Study 202). A natural history cohort of 42 evaluable patients from a DEM-CHILD database was used as the historical control arm (Study 901). The study information is summarized in Table 4.5.

Without widely accepted and objective endpoints for this type of disease, the endpoint in this study was based on the CLN2 rating scale. This

TABLE 4.5

List of Relevant Clinical Studies

Study ID	Phase and Design	Study Population	Treatment Arm(s)	Number of Subjects	Duration
190–901	Non-treatment natural history control cohort based on registry data	Any child diagnosed with a type of neuronal ceroid lipofuscinosis (NCL; including CLN2) that has been confirmed through genetic testing	Do not apply	Overall: 69 Evaluable: 42	Range: 2–61 months (based on data entered in DEM-CHILD database)
190–201	Phase 1/2, first-in-human, single-arm, open-label, dose-escalation	Children ≥3 years old with mild to moderate CLN2 disease, and a baseline Motor-Language summary score of ≥3 (with a score of at least 1 in each of the Motor and Language domains)	ICV infusion every 8 weeks: • 30 mg • 100 mg • Stable dose	Enrolled: 24 Completed: 23	Stable dose treatment period: 48 weeks
190–202	Treatment extension study for subjects who completed 190-201		ICV infusion every 8 weeks: 300 mg	23	Stable dose treatment extension period: up to 240 weeks

unique CLN2 rating scale brought more challenges to the treatment effect evaluation. First, the comparability of the CLN2 rating scale between the natural history cohort control Study 901 and the treatment Studies 201/202 should be carefully assessed because these studies were not conducted at the same time; therefore, the definition of the scales may be different. Second, each patient in Studies 201/202 was rated by only one clinician at each assessment timepoint during the trial. Each subsequent assessment throughout the trial may have been reviewed by a different study clinician. This approach posed potential problems for the evaluation of inter-rater reliability. Third, CLN2 rating assessments were not conducted at regular intervals in Study 901, so the assessment method could be different for the same patient across the study. Therefore, Clinical Outcome Assessment (COA) was based on two parts. The first part was to evaluate the safety, tolerability, PK, and efficacy of Brineura® (which is the common process), and the second part was to assess the adequacy of the CLN2 rating scale and comparability of the scale between the treatment arm and natural history external control arm.

For COA, the CLN2 rating scale is introduced, followed by a discussion about its comparability. The full-length version of the CLN2 rating scale was a clinician-reported outcome (ClinRO) measure that consists of four domains: Motor, Language, Visual, and Seizures. Table 4.6 presents the anchor point definitions for each of the four domains. In this trial, a Motor and Language (ML) total score (ranging from 0 to 6) was reported by summing up the Motor domain score and Language domain score. However, as can be seen from the table, Study 901 and Studies 201/202 used two different versions of the CLN2 rating assessment guidance, which may have resulted in a CLN2 rating scale comparability problem. Treatment effect may be confounded by the different rating scale between Study 901 and Study 201/201 but not the drug effect. Therefore, the Health Authority (i.e., FDA) requested that the applicant submit a full evidence dossier, including analyses to evaluate the CLN2 rating scale comparability between the natural history control and the treatment studies. The agency preferred to rescore all the videotapes of Study 901 patients by the Study 201/202 clinicians, but this was not feasible due to the video availability of historical data and patient privacy laws. Due to language assessment issues and privacy laws, the applicant only conducted analyses using a subset of videos ($n = 71$) from one participating site in Study 201/202. Because each patient was rated by only one clinician at each timepoint in Study 201/202, additional evaluations also were needed for the selected videos. Thus, the strength of agreement between (1) the original rating by the Study 201/202 clinician, (2) the rescoring by the Study 201/202 trainer, and (3) the rescoring by Study 901 CLN2 scale developer were assessed by a graphical approach, weighted kappa, and contingency tables.

Table 4.7 summarized the weighted kappa across all videos and by assessment timepoint for Motor domain, Language domain, and total score. The

TABLE 4.6

CLN2 Rating Scale – Full-Length Version

		Hamburg Scale	
		Study 901	Study 201/202
Motor	3	Walks normally	Grossly normal gait. No prominent ataxia, no pathologic falls.
	2	Frequent falls, obvious clumsiness	Independent gait, as defined by the ability to walk without support for 10 steps. Will have obvious instability, and may have intermittent falls.
	1	No unaided walking or crawling only	Requires external assistance to walk, or can crawl only.
	0	Immobile, mostly bedridden	Can no longer walk or crawl.
Language	3	Normal	Apparently normal language. Intelligible and grossly age appropriate. No decline noted yet.
	2	Recognizably abnormal	Language has become recognizably abnormal: some intelligible words, may form short sentences to convey concepts, requests, or needs. This score signifies a decline from a previous level of ability (from the individual maximum reached by the child).
	1	Hardly understandable	Hardly understandable. Few intelligible words.
	0	Unintelligible or no language	No intelligible words or vocalizations.
Visual	3	Recognizes desirable object, grabs at it	
	2	Grabbing for objects uncoordinated	
	1	Reacts to light	
	0	No reaction to visual stimuli	
Seizures	3	No seizure in 3 months	
	2	1–2 seizures in 3 months	
	1	1 seizure per month	
	0	>1 seizure per month	

criteria of weighted kappa suggested by Landis and Koch (1977) helps to interpret the degree of agreement between different raters.

- < 0.00 = poor agreement
- 0.00–0.20 = slight agreement
- 0.21–0.40 = fair agreement

TABLE 4.7

Summary of Weighted Kappa Across All Videos and by Assessment Timepoint

CLN2 Scale Comparability Study		Motor Domain	Language Domain	ML Total Score
Comparison Strata		Weighted Kappa	Weighted Kappa	Weighted Kappa
Study 201/202 clinician (via "live" assessment)	Study 201/202 trainer (via 36 video assessments)	Overall: 0.93 Baseline: 0.76 201 Week 25: 1.00 201 Completion: 1.00 202 Week 25: 1.00	Overall: 0.82 Baseline: 0.93 201 Week 25: 0.79 201 Completion: 0.67 202 Week 25: 0.80	Overall: 0.92 Baseline: 0.92 201 Week 25: 0.93 201 Completion: 0.89 202 Week 25: 0.93
Study 201/202 clinician (via "live" assessment)	Study 901 CLN2 developer (via 43 video assessments)	Overall: 0.88 Baseline: 0.67 201 Week 25: 0.92 201 Completion: 1.00 202 Week 25: 0.90	Overall: 0.53 Baseline: 0.57 201 Week 25: 0.55 201 Completion: 0.34 202 Week 25: 0.62	Overall: 0.74 Baseline: 0.67 201 Week 25: 0.78 201 Completion: 0.69 202 Week 25: 0.79
Study 901 CLN2 developer (via 36 video assessments)	Study 201/202 trainer (via 36 video assessments)	Overall: 0.94 Baseline: 0.91 201 Week 25: 0.90 201 Completion: 1.00 202 Week 25: 1.00	Overall: 0.56 Baseline: 0.59 201 Week 25: 0.50 201 Completion: 0.48 202 Week 25: 0.67	Overall: 0.82 Baseline: 0.82 201 Week 25: 0.77 201 Completion: 0.80 202 Week 25: 0.88

- 0.41–0.60 = moderate agreement
- 0.61–0.80 = substantial agreement
- 0.81–1.00 = almost agreement

The summarized results showed that ML total score weighted kappa suggested substantial agreement to almost agreement. However, if the results are looked at separately, we see that the Motor domain has a much higher rater agreement compared with the Language domain in terms of overall and at each timepoint. This relatively lower agreement indicated potential problems in the comparability of endpoints between the active drug arms to the historical control arm. The weighted kappa results for the ML total score should be interpreted with caution, as the higher weighted kappa statistic may be dominated by the higher rater agreement observed in the Motor domain component of the total score.

Graphical evaluations and contingency tables also support similar conclusions. The agreement of the Motor domain is strong, but the rates of the Language domain are likely to have inconsistent issues. Based on the CLN2 scale comparability analyses, the COA statistical reviewer concluded that the applicant submitted supportive evidence not sufficiently strong regarding the CLN2 rating scale comparability between the external control Study 901 and the treatment Study 201/202. Based on the evaluation of CLN2 rating consistency analysis, the agency suggested to focus on the Motor domain only.

The efficacy analyses were performed on two analysis populations, based on the different selection criteria of Study 201/202. Table 4.8 shows that the sex and decade born were not well balanced between study 901 and 201/202

TABLE 4.8

Summary of Demographic and Baseline Characteristics

	Study 901 (n = 42)	Study 201/202 Population 1 (n = 22)	Study 201/202 Population 2 (n = 24)
Sex			
Male	25 (60%)	7 (32%)	9 (37.5%)
Female	17 (40%)	15 (68%)	15 (62.5%)
Genotype			
2 key mutations	24 (57%)	9 (41%)	9 (38%)
1 key mutation	11 (26%)	6 (27%)	8 (33%)
No key Mutation	7 (17%)	7 (32%)	7 (29%)
Decade Born			
Pre-1980	4 (10%)	0	0
1980s	2 (5%)	0	0
1990s	19 (45%)	0	0
2000s	16 (38%)	12 (55%)	13 (54%)
≥2010	1 (2%)	10 (45%)	11 (46%)

but were similar between the two populations for studies 201/202. Therefore, the analyses performed were primarily based on population 1.

The primary efficacy analysis is based on a key-variable-matched data set to account for the unbalanced baseline covariates. Key variables, including baseline Motor score, age ± 3 months, and genotype were used to match 22 subjects from Study 201/202 with 42 subjects from Study 901. Table 4.9 summarizes the analyses results. At week 96 follow-up, the difference in response rate is huge and significant.

Other analyses were also performed, including time to decline, ordinal analysis, and binary logistic regression. Given that this is not a standard

TABLE 4.9

Summary of Proportion of Patients (Responder: Unreversed 2-Category Decline or Score of Zero in Motor Domain)

		Study 901 (Natural History) (n = 17)	Study 201/202 (Brineura®) (n = 17)	Difference	Odds Ratio
Response rate *n* **(%)**	Follow-up through Week 48	13 (76%)	16 (94%)	18% (−19, 51)	0.25 (0.005, 2.53)
	Follow-up through Week 72	11 (65%)	16 (94%)	29% (−7, 61)	0.17 (0.004, 1.37)
	Follow-up through Week 96	6 (35%)	16 (94%)	59% (24, 83)	0.09 (0.002, 0.63)

TABLE 4.10

Summary of Other Performed Analyses

Type of Analysis	Model	Hazard Ratio/ Odds Ratio	95% CI
Time-to-unreversed 2-category decline or unreversed score of zero in Motor domain	Covariates: screening baseline age, screening Motor score, and genotype	HR: 0.141	(0.02,1.14)
Ordinal Motor score defined as 0, 1, 2 and 3.	Covariates: screening baseline age, and genotype	OR: 0.17	(0.05,0.6)
Binary logistic regression	Covariates: screening baseline age, screening Motor score, and genotype	OR: 0.08	(0.007,0.86)

randomized clinical trial, Cox regressions were performed adjusting for key covariates including baseline age, baseline screening motor score, and genotype. Results are summarized in Table 4.10. All the statistical analyses confirmed the treatment effect.

In this example, we have seen the challenge of the comparability of endpoints in the rare disease development process. One must take this into account in the design stage. More detailed discussion will be included in Section 4.4.2.

4.2.3 Bavencio® for Patients with Metastatic Merkel Cell Carcinoma (MCC)

The use of historical data as external control was shown to be useful in two rare disease cases. In oncology therapeutic areas, patients with unmet medical needs are also hoping to see promising drugs available on the market faster. Many accelerated approval drugs were based on single-arm trials with objective overall response rate (ORR) as the endpoint (FDA 2018b). Finding a reference ORR to compare with the single-arm trial depends on the specific disease and number of lines of treatment a patient has received. Sometimes an objective reference level derived from RWD or historical control is helpful to make the fair comparison.

In 2017, the FDA approved Bavencio® (avelumab) as a treatment for adults and pediatric patients 12 years and older with metastatic MCC under the Accelerated Approval regulations (FDA 2017b). The primary analysis supporting the clinical efficacy and safety evidence of Bavencio® in patients with metastatic MCC comes from Study 003, a single-arm trial with 88 patients. For the primary efficacy endpoint, confirmed best ORR was 33%, with 95% confidence interval (CI) (23%, 44%). Further details are shown in Table 4.11 The secondary efficacy endpoint is duration of response (DOR), which ranges from 2.8 months to 23.3 months (ongoing). The Kaplan-Meier estimate for the percentage of patients with a 6-month DOR is 93% (95% CI: 74%, 98%), and the estimate for the percentage of patients with a 12-month DOR is 75% (95% CI: 53%, 87%).

TABLE 4.11

Summary of response of Study 003

Type of Analysis	Avelumab ($N = 88$) n (%)
Confirmed Responses	29 (33.0%)
Complete Responses	10 (11.4%)
Partial Responses	19 (21.6%)
Stable Disease	9 (10.2%)
Progressive Disease	32 (36.4%)
Not evaluable	18 (20.5%)

The efficacy results of Study 003 were compared with Study Obs001, which was a retrospective chart review and registry-based study. In this study, 686 patients in the United States were identified in the iKnow Med electronic health record database. According to disease types, follow-up times, and prior treatment, 14 patients defined as immunocompetent were identified as the reference group. This group of patients most closely mimicked the Study 003 population. The ORR in these 14 patients was 28.6% (95% CI: 8.4, 58.1), with a median DOR of 1.7 months (95% CI: 0.5, 3.0). The key variables matched in the analysis only focused on the underlying disease, without considering demographic variables due to the limited number of subjects. Compared with the efficacy results in Study 003, moderate improvement was noted in the ORR and huge improvement in the DOR.

In this example, the matching procedure is based only on a few variables and a small number of patients from registry data. Therefore, this external control arm is only considered as supportive evidence given the limitation of the historical data. Even so, for a serious and life-threatening disease for which there is no FDA-approved therapy and no known curative therapy, the historical control arm provides an objective reference level to with which to compare. In this example, the comparison of DOR offers supportive evidence, which is very important for a disease with such short DOR under the standard treatment.

4.3 Comparison Across Trials with External Control for Label Expansion

In Section 4.2, we reviewed how to use an external control arm in clinical development for an NDA and BLA. In the drug development process, after the first NDA or BLA, a supplemental new drug application (sNDA) or supplemental Biologic License Application (sBLA) may also be applied to expand labels to more indications, patients, or regimens. For oncology drug development, since cancer can be divided into different stages and subtypes, label expansion is a very common way to benefit a broader patient population with the approved drugs. In addition, cancer treatments often adopt various combination treatment regimens, while the initial NDA or BLA may only cover one regimen. Moreover, in clinical practice, some regimens may be used off-label. These clinical practice regimens provide large amounts of RWD and historical data. Therefore, how to adopt these data as external controls for label expansion is also critical in drug development. In this section, two unique examples with different emphasis will be used to illustrate how to use external controls for label expansion. Both examples use the propensity score (PS) method to account for confounding factors due to lack of direct randomization. In this section, only the practical use of the PS method will be discussed. The theoretical details of the PS method will be discussed in later sections (Section 4.4.3 and Section 7). In Section 4.3.1, we will emphasize how to use PS matching (PSM) to construct an external control arm. In Section 4.3.2, we will illustrate how to use inverse probability treatment weighting.

4.3.1 Velcade® Label Expansion for Patients with Relapsed and/or Progressive Multiple Myeloma

Multiple myeloma (MM) is a cancer that forms in a type of white blood cell called a plasma cell. The treatment of MM has changed during the last 10–15 years. With the development of the proteasome inhibitor Velcade® and the immunomodulatory agent Revlimid, Velcade®-dexamethasone (VD)-based and Revlimid-dexamethasone (RD)-based therapies have become the backbone of combination therapy (Rajkumar and Kumar 2016). When Velcade® was approved as a single-agent treatment for relapsed MM, the efficacy and safety profile of Velcade® was characterized in the phase III APEX study and in the phase III DOXIL-MMY-3001 study (Kane et al. 2006). As the other research progressed, results from several clinical trials suggested that adding dexamethasone to bortezomib can improve response rates in patients. The VD doublet regimen was widely used in routine clinical practice for relapsed MM patients in 2013. However, a direct comparison of VD versus Velcade® monotherapy was missing. Therefore, a meaningful cross-study comparison using different adequate arms to compare the VD doublet regimen versus Velcade® monotherapy was needed. The label expansion of Velcade® plus dexamethasone in patients with relapsed and/or progressive MM who have received at least one prior therapy was approved in the European Union (EU) in 2013 (European Medicines Agency [EMA] 2013, Dimopoulos et al. 2015). This approval was based on an integrated analysis that comprised three clinical trials: MMY-2045, APEX, and DOXIL-MMY-3001. The study information is summarized in Table 4.12.

Outcomes were compared using subjects in the VD group from Study MMY-2045 to propensity-score-matched control subjects from the Velcade® monotherapy arms in Study APEX and Study MMY-3001.

TABLE 4.12

Summary of Related Study Information for Velcade® Label Expansion Studies

Studies	Study Design	Treatment Groups	No. of Subjects
MMY-3001	Phase 3 randomized study Primary endpoint: time to progression	Group A: Velcade Group B: Velcade + CAELYX/ DOXIL	Group A: 322 Group B: 324
APEX	Randomized, open-label study in patients with RRMM	Group A: (Velcade) Group B: High-dose dexamethasone	Group A: 333 Group B: 336
MMY-2045	Phase 2	Part 1 (nonrandomized treatment - all subjects): Velcade + Dex Part 2: (subjects with SD were randomized to Group B, C, or D below; subjects with ≥PR continued as in group A) Group B: Velcade + Dex Group C: Velcade + Dex + cyclophosphamide Group D: Velcade + Dex + lenalidomide	Group A: 144 Group B: 7 Group C: 8 Group D: 4

The PSM in this analysis included eight identified variables that were related to clinical outcome: age; Eastern Cooperative Oncology Group (ECOG) score; type of myeloma; percentage of plasma cells; prior dexamethasone; and hemoglobin, creatinine clearance, and albumin. A total of 127 patients were identified in each arm using PSM.

The clinical outcomes were compared using ORR, progression-free survival (PFS), time to progression (TTP), and OS. The ORR in the VD group is significantly higher than that in the Velcade® monotherapy group. The odds ratio with 95% CI was 3.769 (2.045, 6.947). PFS also provided evidence to show clinical benefit for VD. The median PFS was 10.7 months for the VD arm and was 6.2 months for the Velcade® monotherapy group. The hazard ratio for VD versus Velcade® monotherapy was 0.511, with 95% CI (0.309, 0.845), and p-value 0.008.

In this example, the PSM method was performed to match the patients in the external control group. Instead of using several variables in the exact key variable matching procedure, PSM only uses PS as a summary of important variables in the matching procedure. Other PS methods will be introduced in the later sections.

4.3.2 Blincyto® Label Expansion for Minimal Residual Disease Positive (MRD+) Acute Lymphoblastic Leukemia (ALL)

Blincyto®, developed by Amgen, is a bispecific CD19-directed CD3 T-cell engager. The first indication of Blincyto® was to treat relapsed or refractory B-cell precursor ALL in adults and children (Przepiorka et al. 2015). In 2018, the FDA expanded the approval of Blincyto® to treat MRD+ B-cell precursor ALL (FDA 2017a). This sBLA approval was based on a pivotal phase 2, open-label, single-arm study (Study 203) and two supplemental studies, Study 202 and Study 148. In study 203, 116 patients were enrolled and 113 were used in the final analysis.

The primary endpoint of Study 203 was the MRD response rate, which was defined as the incidence of MRD negativity with one cycle of treatment with Blincyto®. The complete MRD response rate within the first cycle was 77.9% (95% CI: 69.1, 85.1), which was significantly greater than the null hypothesis threshold of 44%. Some key secondary analyses included relapse-free survival (RFS) and OS.

A prospectively integrated analysis, which combined Blincyto® active treatment in Study 203 and historical control in Study 148, was conducted to compare RFS and OS. Study 148 was a retrospective non-interventional cohort study of historical treatment and outcome data from MRD-positive patients with Philadelphia-negative B-cell precursor ALL who had received standard-of-care treatment according to national study protocols. Assessment of MRD response was not included in the study because of the variability in treatment regimens after documentation of MRD-positive status. The purpose of this study was to estimate RFS and OS and compare them to the Blincyto® treatment arm in Study 203. Among the total 287 patients in the final analysis set in Study 148, 182 patients were selected for the integrated analysis with Study 203, based on similar inclusion criteria. Adding a criterion of a minimum of 14 days between MRD measurement and start of blinatumomab further reduced the sample size in the blinatumomab arm (Study 203) from 113 to 73. This more than 30% reduction of sample size in the treatment arm can reduce the power and may cause selection bias.

The inverse probability of treatment weighting (IPTW) method was used to adjust the covariate balance. This method adopted PS as a weight for each patient and calculated the weighted treatment effect. To estimate the PS for the patient in the logistic regression, several covariates were identified. The majority of the covariates were chosen based on prognostic factors that have been identified for ALL in published literature and to account for potential regional differences in treatment practices. They are

- Age at primary diagnosis (years)
- Sex (male, female)
- Country (Germany, others)
- Presence and type of any cytogenetic and molecular aberrations
- Time from primary diagnosis to MRD baseline date (months)
- Baseline MRD level
- White blood cell (WBC) count at diagnosis
- Type of prior chemotherapy (GMALL, other)

RFS and OS were analyzed using a weighted Cox proportional hazards regression with robust variance estimation with 95% CIs around the resulting hazard ratio for the treatment covariate. For RFS, the hazard ratio is 0.50 with 95% CI: 0.32, 0.78, which is a significant result indicating the treatment effect of Blincyto®. The Kaplan-Meier (KM)-based median RFS, unadjusted for hematopoietic stem cell transplantation (HSCT), was estimated at 8.3 months (95% CI: 6.2, 11.8) for control and 35.2 months (95% CI: 24.2, not evaluable (NE)) for Blincyto®. For OS, the hazard ratio is 0.76 (95% CI: 0.47, 1.24), which is not significant. The KM-based median OS, unadjusted for HSCT, was estimated at 27.2 months (95% CI: 16.4, 38.6) for control and 36.5 months (95% CI: 24.2, NE) for Blincyto®.

This analysis using PS demonstrated that the RFS with blinatumomab was significantly greater than the historical controls, but the sponsor and FDA also recognized some limitations:

- Although the PS method balanced the selected covariates, there are uncertainties for unmeasured or unknown covariates. If some of the important covariates were not in the PS model, they can be potential confounding factors.
- The analysis was based on a subgroup of the treatment arm. More than 30% of the patients in the treatment arm were excluded in analyses, which may lead to selection bias and a reduction in statistical power.
- The follow-up time between the blinatumomab group and historical control group was not comparable.

4.4 Important Considerations When Designing Studies and Analyzing Data Using External Control in Clinical Development

4.4.1 Study Selection

To mimic randomized clinical trials and reduce bias, subjects in two arms must have similar baseline characteristics. More specifically, a valid external control from RWD or a historical study should have the similar eligibility requirements, inclusion and exclusion criteria, medical conditions, and clinical evaluations as the active arm. This way, patients in the external arm will mimic patients from the clinical trial and thus closely resemble the treatment arm in all known relevant baseline variables including disease severity, duration of illness, prior treatments, and any other variables that affect outcomes and treatments. Having comparable clinical evaluations and outcomes in each group is also very important. Otherwise, bias exists when estimating treatment effect. Therefore, identifying such an external control arm with adequate RWD and/or historical study is critical for designing a study. In practice, however, selecting an adequate external control arm may not be easy. First, finding the relevant historical studies and RWD that have similar characteristics could be difficult. One may think the RWD or historical data would be massive in this "big data" era. However, when considering all the factors, including inclusion criteria, exclusion criteria, disease severity, duration of illness, prior treatments, and endpoints, the eligible similar studies may still be limited. Second, even if one can find similar studies, getting access to the patient-level data from these studies may also be challenging due to the platform or privacy restriction. Finally, the data quality of RWD and historical data may be another concern due to reasons like missing data, criteria change, and standard medical condition change.

In the examples reviewed in this chapter, we have seen several successful examples that adopted an external control in drug development. Among them, natural history studies were often used to support rare diseases NDAs and BLAs. The FDA (2019a) recently released a new guidance for rare diseases: Natural History Studies for Drug Development for Industry. This guidance provides information about the design and implementation of natural history studies that can be used to support the development of safe and effective drugs and biological products for rare diseases. On the other hand, for oncology label expansion examples reviewed in this chapter, cross-study comparisons were commonly used. Cross-studies often include one novel label expansion arm and a historical control arm, which can be the standard of care or the regimen containing the first approved indication of the applied drug. Unlike natural history studies used in the rare disease examples, historical data from previous clinical trials that were conducted by the same or different sponsors can be used. Data from investigator-initiated sponsored trials or data-sharing platforms also can be used as the external control.

We also have seen the trend of using registry and electronic record data for the application. In the Bavencio® example that we reviewed, the efficacy of the Bavencio® arm was compared with Study Obs001, which is a retrospective chart review and registry-based study. In April 2019, Ibrance® (developed by Pfizer) was approved by the FDA for a new indication. This label expansion of Ibrance in combination with an aromatase inhibitor or fulvestrant to include men with certain types of metastatic breast cancer was based on RWD from electronic health records and post-marketing data (Pfizer 2019). RWD in this study were extracted from three databases: IQVIA insurance database, Flatiron Health Breast Cancer database, and Pfizer Global Safety database. In addition, some commercial data service companies are also building a data-sharing platform. Corroborating with research centers, hospitals, and industry, data from these sources can be integrated and stored in the platform. If one would like to compare a new treatment to a standard of care, a synthetic control arm can be extracted from the data set. The synthetic control arm will mimic a randomized, controlled clinical trial with baseline characteristics similar to the treatment arm. In a white paper, Davie et al. (2018) demonstrated that it is possible to produce "matched" cohorts of patients from historical clinical trials using PSs derived from observed baseline characteristics with a non-small cell lung cancer (NSCLC) example. The OS outcome results of the synthetic control were observed to be very similar to that of the control arm in the randomized clinical trial.

In the big data era, researchers are not short of data. The important issue is how to select the right RWD and historical data to generate RWE that can be adequately used in the clinical development. Even after finding the adequate data, there are many practical considerations for how to use and analyze them.

4.4.2 Comparability of Data

In all the reviewed examples in this chapter, guaranteeing the comparability of data is very important. Patients' baseline characteristics and endpoint measurements for the treatment group and the control group should be similar for fair comparison. Without comparability between groups in terms of baseline covariates and outcome measurement, the estimation of treatment effect is biased, so the results cannot be used in the confirmatory trials.

For rare diseases, the limited number of patients and limited knowledge of the diseases bring a great deal of challenges to clinical trial design. Sufficient patients and covariates to fit logistic regression is required to use PSMs. With limited patients (often less than 100 patients) in the rare disease trials, PSM may not be able to match enough similar patients, which will lower the statistical power. Therefore, matching based on some key variables that are correlated to the disease outcomes is commonly used. The limitation of this key variables exact matching is the potential unbalances in other unmatched variables. Moreover, if the disease has not been deeply researched and thoroughly understood, even the endpoints of the trials could be hard to determine. We have seen different ways to define CLN2 rating in Section 4.2.2 and how to check the comparability of the different measurements. This procedure required extensive work. The Health Authority suggested scheduling a meeting with them as early as possible to discuss the choice of endpoints to make sure endpoints from the current study and historical data will be comparable. If a well-defined endpoint is used, for example, OS, it reduces the uncertainty of consistency when comparing the active treatment arm to control arms, which are derived from RWD or other types of historical data.

For oncology studies, even with a relatively larger sample size, there are still some challenges. The treatment of oncology can be divided into many lines, which reflects the different stages of disease for patients. Therefore, the comparison between the novel oncology treatment regimen and the standard of care or old treatment has to make sure that patient populations are comparable between the two arms. Finding similar studies conducted by the same sponsor, cancer center, and research center could help to target the right population. When using the RWD, one must use the same inclusion and exclusion as in the treatment arm to select the historical control patients. Once the right target populations or trials are selected, one can use key variables or PSMs to mimic the randomization. The endpoints of oncology studies – such as OS, PFS, and ORR – are quite objective. However, endpoints based on tumor assessment such as PFS or ORR may use different criteria or versions. One must be careful when evaluating the endpoints in the control arm, because they may have been derived on the basis of old version criteria compared with the active treatment arm. Adopting independent verification or judication of the assessment for both arms could contribute to the consistency of the endpoints. In addition, time-to-event (TTE) type endpoints may bring extra challenges because (1) follow-up time can vary a great deal from study to study, which affects the availability of summary statistics, and (2) potential subsequent therapies, which sometimes can contribute, prolong OS considerably.

4.4.3 Methods for PS Model

The PS method (Rosenbaum and Rubin 1983) was used to mimic randomized clinical trial in the analysis. When direct randomization is lacking, the outcome differences may be attributed to unbalanced covariates but not the treatment effect. The PS method can contribute to balance covariates between two arms and make the quasi-randomization set. Because the study is not a randomized clinical trial, using PS approaches helps to reduce confounding bias due to lack of randomization. PS is, given an observed set of covariates, what is the probability of having a certain outcome or be assigned to a certain treatment. Some mathematical notations for PSs are as follows:

- Treatment assignment: $Z_i = 1$ if subject i was in the treated group; $Z_i = 0$ if subject i is in the control group
- Observed covariates: X
- Outcomes: $Y_i(1)$ is the outcome for subject i if he or she was assigned to the treated group; $Y_i(0)$ is the outcome for subject i if he or she was assigned to the control group
- The formal mathematical definition of PS is $e(X_i) = \Pr(Z_i = 1 | X_i)$.

If these assumptions hold, the treatment assignment is ignorable. Therefore, conditioning on the PS allows us to obtain an unbiased average treatment effect. If two PSs are similar, it means they have the same probability to be assigned to the same treatment group and their characteristics are similar. If they are in the different groups, it mimics the randomization; the outcome difference only attributes to the treatment effect, not other lurking variables.

4.4.3.1 Matching by PS

PSM is one of the PS methods that reduces the imbalance of covariates. The main idea of PSM is to match treated and untreated subjects who share similar values of the PS to create a quasi-randomization set. The 1:1 matching is most often used. In some cases, however, such as more subjects in the comparison group or the limited number of subjects in the treatment group, 1:n matching also can be used.

There are several PSM methods (D'Agostino 1998, Rosenbaum 2010). Most of them can be categorized into two major algorithms, greedy matching and optimal matching. In greedy matching, a subject in the treated group is selected randomly, then a subject in the control group who has the nearest PS is matched with the picked subject in the treated group. This matching process is repeated until all subjects are matched. Instead of reducing the divergences of PSs between each pair, optimal matching, on the other hand, minimizes the global distance measure of total matched pairs.

Optimal matching is often used with a pre-specified caliper. For a given treated subject, we would identify all the untreated subjects whose PSs are within a specified distance of that of the treated subject. Then, the matching is processed. If no untreated subjects have PSs that are within the specified caliper distance of the PS of the treated subject that treated subject would not be matched with any untreated subjects. The unmatched treated subject would, therefore, be excluded from the matched sample.

4.4.3.2 Stratification by PS

Unlike the PSM method that only selected subjects with similar PSs, stratification by propensity could include all the PS-available subjects. By using all subjects who are PS available, subjects are stratified into mutually exclusive subsets based on their estimated PSs. For this method, PS values are used as a stratification factor. The method follows these steps:

1. PS is estimated by logistic regression.
2. Look at quintiles of the estimated PS.
3. Decide cutoff points for different strata.
4. Compare outcome difference within stratum.
5. Estimate overall treatment effect.

Normally, samples are stratified into five approximately equal-size quintiles based on estimated PS; this removes 90% of the bias of the covariates, as described by Rosenbaum and Rubin (1984).

4.4.3.3 IPTW

An IPTW was also performed in the analysis. Individuals are weighted by the inverse probability of receiving the treatment as assigned/randomized. The basic idea is to use the PS as a weight variable. The weight for treatment patient is $\frac{1}{e_i}$, and the weight for control patient is $\frac{1}{1-e_i}$. They can be rewritten as $w_i = \frac{Z_i}{e_i} + \frac{(1-Z_i)}{1-e_i}$.

The IPTW method is also inclusive of all PS-available subjects. A drawback of the IPTW method is the possibility of extreme PSs that can result in very large weights. Possible solutions are (1) stabilize the weights with the mean for each treatment group and (2) exclude these patients.

These three methods can be used in the study design and outcome analysis for confirmatory trials, because the design part and outcome analysis part can be separated. During the first part, the PS model can be constructed with baseline covariates only. Outcome data are masked in the first part. Once the PS model in the first part is constructed, one can estimate treatment effect using outcome data.

4.4.3.4 Another Example Using Stratification by PS

Similar to the VD example for patients with relapsed, refractory MM (RRMM) in the previous section, in oncology clinical practice combination regimens sometimes can be used off-label before the formal label expansion application is submitted to the Health Authority. Combination treatment A was a popular and useful triplet regimen for MM patients, but there were no formal randomized clinical trials to directly compare the treatment effect of treatment A with all the standard of care. One of the main reasons for lacking such a formal randomized clinical trial to support the label expansion is the ethical issue. Because several previous studies have already shown the clinical benefits to patients from using the combination regimen A, it would be unethical to prevent patients in a standard-of-care control group from using regimen A. In addition, it is not feasible to conduct such a new clinical trial because patients in the control group may drop the study and switch to other novel combination treatments. Even with these challenges, there is still a need for a cross-study comparison to support label expansion and to compare the clinical benefit of combination regimen A with the standard of care.

Patient-level data were available for combination regimen A from clinical trial I and for standard-of-care regimen B from clinical trial II. The analysis was based on cross-study comparisons using these two clinical trials. Stratification by the PS method was used for the efficacy analyses. Unlike the PSM method, which only selects subjects with similar PSs, stratification by propensity includes all the PS-available subjects.

This approach makes full use of PS-evaluable subjects and increases the power of the analysis. Other PS methods, including IPTW, matching by PS, and regression also were examined. Detailed results are summarized in Section 4.4.5.

4.4.4 Methods for Baseline Covariate Selection and Checking

The assumptions of the PS method rely highly on no unmeasured confounders. In the ideal situation, all the variables should be included in the PS model because it makes use of all the available information to avoid unknown confounders. Some researchers have concerns about the unmeasured confounders' assumptions when the external control arm is used in real clinical practice. In reality, one cannot collect all the variables and use them in the PS model because nobody could completely define "all variables" for a patient. In addition, the PS for a subject is evaluable only if there are no missing baseline covariate values for this subject. If one of the important variables is missing for a subject, the PS for this subject could not be estimated. Thus, the sample size of the PS population will be smaller and lead to selection bias and lower statistical power. To select the important covariates in the PS model, people often rely on clinical relevance, literature reviews, statistical models, or a hybrid of these methods.

Based on medical and biological knowledge, one can identify candidate variables that either affect the outcomes or treatment assignments. For well-researched diseases, publications from the previous studies also will provide some important insights on covariate identification. With this information, one can include all the covariates through clinical inputs and literature reviews or select some of them based on statistical modeling. Some model selection tools include Akaike information criterion (AIC), Bayesian information criterion (BIC), and stepwise regression selection. For rare diseases or other less well-known diseases, there would be limited information for covariate selection. In this situation, many baseline covariates can be candidate variables for the PS model. Sometimes, the number of variables may exceed the number of subjects. In this scenario, modern statistical learning methods including least absolute shrinkage and selection operator (LASSO), or random forest–based model selection tools, can be used to select the covariates used in the PS model.

Another concern of using RWE or other forms of data as historical control is study population differences. Without a strict randomized clinical trial, one cannot guarantee patients in the two groups are similar. Therefore, before demonstrating the efficacy benefit of the new drugs or new indication, providing the evidence of baseline covariate balance is critical.

For the exact variables matching method using some key variables, reporting descriptive statistics and/or standard difference is helpful to show whether the baseline variables are balanced or not. For deceptive statistics, mean with standard deviation (SD), median, min, and max are commonly reported for continuous variables. Numbers and percentages are often reported for categorical variables.

When the sample size is larger and the number of baseline variables needed to report is larger, the standardized difference is commonly used. The standardized difference compares the difference in means in units of the pooled SD, and it allows for the comparison of the relative balance of variables measured in different units. This method also avoids multiple comparisons when we just simply use the t-test. The standardized difference provides a framework for comparing the mean or prevalence of a baseline covariate between two treatment groups. A standardized difference less than 0.1 indicates a negligible difference in means between two groups (Austin and Mamdani 2006).

- Continuous variable: $d = \dfrac{\bar{x}_{\text{treated}} - \bar{x}_{\text{control}}}{\sqrt{\dfrac{s^2_{\text{treated}} + s^2_{\text{control}}}{2}}}$

- Dichotomous variable: $d = \dfrac{\hat{p}_{\text{treated}} - \hat{p}_{\text{control}}}{\sqrt{\dfrac{\hat{p}_{\text{treated}}(1 - \hat{p}_{\text{treated}}) - \hat{p}_{\text{control}}(1 - \hat{p}_{\text{control}})}{2}}}$

In the example reviewed in Section 4.4.3.4, before stratification by PS, 3 of 11 variables were not balanced, and after stratification by PS, all the variables used in the PS model were balanced. Under this covariate well-balanced assumption, any subsequent outcomes comparison becomes more fair and trustworthy.

In addition to the reporting descriptive statistics and standard difference to compare covariate balance, other forms of comparisons can also be used when the PS-related method is used. The fundamental step of checking PS performances is to check the PS distributions using a histogram or boxplot. Only if the PS distributions for two groups have enough overlapping area can we start to use PS for the rest of the analysis. (Austin 2011a&b)

Specifically, for PS matching, we need to check the PS distribution after matching between two groups. For PS stratification, we also need to check PS distributions across strata between two groups. The first and last stratum should be checked with more attention, because all extreme PS values would be included in these two strata.

Figure 4.1 shows that the PSs between two groups were comparable in terms of shape, mean, min, and max values. Similar trends also can be seen in Figure 4.2, when stratification is performed using PSs.

One can also use a regression model to check the covariate balance before and after stratification by PS (Rosenbaum and Rubin 1984). The difference in mean covariate values across strata will be compared between the two cohorts using a regression model, with covariate as the dependent variable. For a continuous variable, the standard linear regression will be used. For a categorical variable, the logistic regression will be used. The summary results

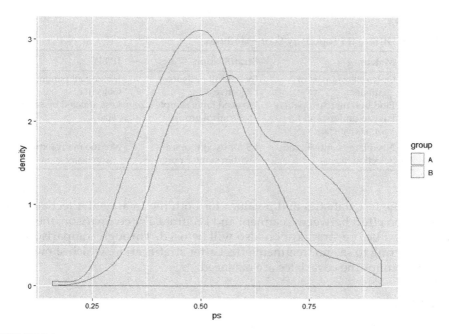

FIGURE 4.1
Propensity score distribution.

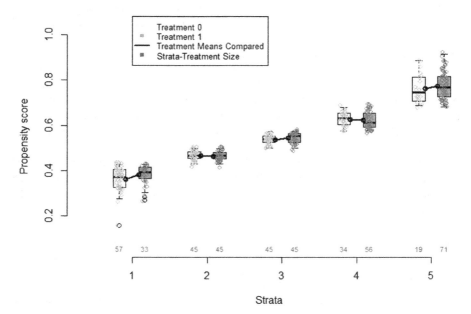

FIGURE 4.2
Propensity score distribution by stratum.

TABLE 4.13

Compare Different Propensity Score Methods

Methods	Matching	Stratification	IPTW
Pros	Only selected part of patients Find best matched patients Easy to understand for non-statistician	Include all patients Objective No need large sample size for control group	Include all patients Objective Less affected by sample size
Cons	Need large control group Selection bias	PS for two groups are within similar range	Not too many extreme propensity score values

contain the test statistics and p-values for both the treatment effect and the interaction effect between treatment and PS strata. For comparison, the treatment effect before stratification also will be used. Through comparison, we are expecting to see no treatment effect after stratification, which shows that for two groups the covariates are balanced.

4.4.5 Sensitivity Analysis

Given considerable concerns about using external controls in the analyses, the Health Authority may require different types of sensitivity analyses to make sure the results are robust. Some common concerns, as described in previous sections, are comparability of endpoints, baseline variables used in the matching or in the PS model, model assumption, and missing data. The comparability of endpoints was discussed in Section 4.4.2. This section will focus on the sensitivity analysis related to PS methods.

Let us start by comparing the different PS methods that are summarized in Table 4.13. Often one PS method may be used as the primary analysis method. However, due to the limitations of each method, additional analyses based on other PS methods also will be performed. Li et al. (2020) also summarized additional information on practical considerations of utilizing PS methods in clinical development.

A PS method can be affected by (1) missing values, (2) number of variables used in the model, (3) unobserved covariates, and (4) tuning parameters in the matching procedure. Therefore, it is also important to conduct sensitivity analyses to demonstrate the robustness of the results. The following sensitivity analyses are helpful:

- *Imputation of missing baseline variables*: There are several ways to impute missing values. For continuous variables, mean or median can be used. For categorical variables, we can randomly assign a number using the distribution parameters calculated by the complete cases. Further, the worst or the best risk categories can be assigned to the missing variables, to assess the effect in extreme cases.

- *Changing variables used in the model*: Number of variables included in the PS estimation model can be explored to further check the impact of changing variables in the models to the treatment effects and model assumption.
- *Changing caliper or exact matching variables for matching*: changing caliper in the procedure will filter the number of matched subjects in the control group. A tight caliper may reduce bias by using the strict criteria, but some subjects could not be matched. A loose caliper will increase the number of matched pairs. Similarly, if the number of exact matching variables increase, matched subjects should be much more similar, but may result in less qualified subjects.
- *Covariate adjusted regression*: Covariates used in the regression can also be changed. Like changing the number of variables in the PS model, we can add or reduce the number of variables used in the regression model. One way is to use all the variables without missing values, it helps to increase the sample size.

Figure 4.3 summarizes all the standard analysis and sensitivity analysis results in Section 4.4.3. The endpoint is ORR. As seen from the figure, results

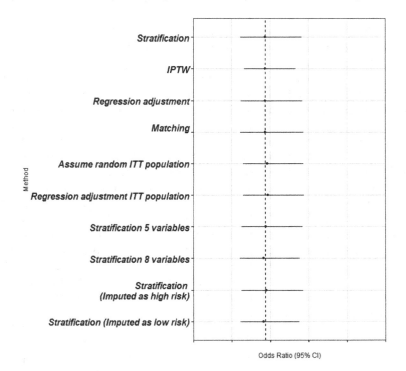

FIGURE 4.3
Summary of analysis results.

were consistent across different analysis methods and sensitivity analyses using different assumptions. These results demonstrated the robustness of the results.

4.4.6 Prospectively Plan and Objectively Study Design

Because using RWD and historical data as external controls has many practical considerations, the Health Authority recommends a prospectively defined statistical analysis plan (SAP). The SAP should include the analysis population, definition of endpoints, deceptive objectives, testable hypothesis, and statistical methods. The integrity of the analysis also should be carefully executed. It is critical to prospectively plan the use of RWD/historical data and objectively design a study for the evaluation of the confirmatory trials. During the design stage, clinical outcome variables from RWD/historical data should not be analyzed to avoid data dredging. The design stage must be outcome free to mimic the prospective randomized clinical trials.

Specifically, for studies that use PS modeling, the rules of how to select baseline covariates should be clearly defined in the SAP. One must establish the PS model and estimate the individual PS before getting access to the outcome data. Analyzing outcome data before constructing a PS model should be avoided to protect the objectives and integrity of the analyses. If PSM is used, the random seed also needs to be recorded in the analysis because there could be randomness in the pairing process.

In practice, PS modeling may not be completely well defined in the SAP due to some unexpected uncertainties. For example, the PS value for a patient is evaluable only if there are no missing baseline values for this patient. If a specific variable defined in the SAP has many missing values, then the PS model cannot be constructed successfully. Given this challenge, we have to admit that PS modeling is an iterative process that cannot be fully pre-specified. In cases like this, an independent statistician who builds PS models without outcome data could help maintain the integrity.

A design using external control can be divided into two stages. The first stage is initial planning of a study by the sponsor. At this stage, the sponsor plans the study as in a randomized clinical trial. At the same time, one can identify an independent design statistician, who is blinded from the outcome data, to help build a firewall to mask the outcome data for both treated and control arm patients. After the patients in the treated arm have been enrolled, the second stage should start. Based on the patient population in the treatment group, one can select a comparable external control group from RWD and other historical studies. The independent statistician will build the PS model and examine the covariate balances between the two arms to make sure the populations are comparable. Then, based on different PS modeling, one can specify how to estimate treatment effects in the SAP.

Acknowledgments

We would like to thank Jennifer Tunnicliffe, Takeda Pharmaceuticals, Inc, and Yingying Liu, Biogen, Inc., for editing assistance. Your contributions were a great help for polishing this chapter.

References

21st Century Cures Act. H.R. 34, 114th Congress. 2016. https://www.gpo.gov/fdsys/pkg/BILLS-114hr34enr/pdf/BILLS-114hr34enr.pdf.

Austin, P.C. 2011a. A tutorial and case study in propensity score analysis: an application to estimating the effect of in-hospital smoking cessation counseling on mortality. *Multivariate Behavioral Research*, 46(1), 119–151.

Austin, P.C. 2011b. An introduction to propensity score methods for reducing the effects of confounding in observational studies. *Multivariate Behavioral Research*, 46(3), 399–424.

Austin, P.C. and Mamdani, M.M. 2006. A comparison of propensity score methods: a case-study estimating the effectiveness of post - AMI statin use. *Statistics in Medicine*, 25(12), 2084–2106.

D'Agostino Jr, R.B. 1998. Propensity score methods for bias reduction in the comparison of a treatment to a non-randomized control group. *Statistics in Medicine*, 17(19), 2265–2281.

Davi, R., et al. December 16, 2018. Exploring Whether A Synthetic Control Arm can be Derived from Historical Clinical Trials that Match Baseline Characteristics and Overall Survival Outcome of a Randomized Control Arm. https://www.focr.org/sites/default/files/pdf/SCA%20White%20Paper.pdf

Dimopoulos, M.A., Orlowski, R.Z., Facon, T., Sonneveld, P., Anderson, K.C., Beksac, M., Benboubker, L., et al. 2015. Retrospective matched-pairs analysis of bortezomib plus dexamethasone versus bortezomib monotherapy in relapsed multiple myeloma. *Haematologica*, 100(1), 100–106.

European Medicines Agency [EMA]. 2013. Assessment report: VELCADE: Procedure No. EMEA/H/C/000539/II/0063/G. https://www.ema.europa.eu/en/medicines/human/EPAR/velcade#assessment-history-section

Food and Drug Administration [FDA]. 1998. Guidance for industry: providing clinical evidence of effectiveness for human drug and biological products. https://www.fda.gov/regulatory-information/search-fda-guidance-documents/providing-clinical-evidence-effectiveness-human-drug-and-biological-products

Food and Drug Administration [FDA]. 2014a. Guidance for industry: expedited programs for serious conditions – drugs and biologics. https://www.fda.gov/media/86377/download

Food and Drug Administration [FDA]. 2014b. Guidance for industry: rare diseases: common issues in drug development. https://www.fda.gov/media/119757/download

Food and Drug Administration [FDA]. 2015. Statistical review: application number 125513Orig1s000. https://www.accessdata.fda.gov/drugsatfda_docs/nda/2015/125513Orig1s000MedR.pdf

Food and Drug Administration [FDA]. 2017a. FDA briefing document oncologic drugs advisory committee meeting: BLA 125557 S-013, Blincyto (blinatumomab). https://www.fda.gov/media/111622/download

Food and Drug Administration [FDA]. 2017b. Multi-discipline review: application number 761049Orig1s000. https://www.accessdata.fda.gov/drugsatfda_docs/nda/2017/761049Orig1s000MultidisciplineR.pdf

Food and Drug Administration [FDA]. 2017c. Statistical review: application number 761052Orig1s000. https://www.accessdata.fda.gov/drugsatfda_docs/nda/2017/761052Orig1s000StatR.pdf

Food and Drug Administration [FDA]. 2018a. Framework for FDA's real-world evidence program, 2018. https://www.fda.gov/media/120060/download

Food and Drug Administration [FDA]. 2018b. Guidance for industry: clinical trial endpoints for the approval of cancer drugs and biologics. https://www.fda.gov/media/71195/download

Food and Drug Administration [FDA]. 2019a. Guidance for industry: rare diseases: natural history studies for drug development. https://www.fda.gov/media/122425/download

Food and Drug Administration [FDA]. 2019b. Guidance for industry: submitting documents using real-world data and real-world evidence to FDA for drugs and biologics. https://www.fda.gov/media/124795/download

Kane, R.C., Farrell, A.T., Sridhara, R., and Pazdur, R. 2006. United States Food and Drug Administration approval summary: bortezomib for the treatment of progressive multiple myeloma after one prior therapy. *Clinical Cancer Research,* 12(10), 2955–2960.

Landis, J.R. and Koch, G.G. 1977. The measurement of observer agreement for categorical data. *Biometrics,* 159–174.

Li, Q., Lin, J., Chi, A., & Davies, S. (2020). Practical considerations of utilizing propensity score methods in clinical development using real-world and historical data. Contemporary Clinical Trials, 106123. https://doi.org/10.1016/j.cct.2020.106123

Meldrum, M. L. (2000). A brief history of the randomized controlled trial: From oranges and lemons to the gold standard. *Hematology/oncology clinics of North America,* 14(4), 745–760.

Pfizer. 2019. U.S. FDA approves Ibrance® (palbociclib) for the treatment of men with HR+, HER2- metastatic breast cancer.

Przepiorka, D., Ko, C.W., Deisseroth, A., Yancey, C.L., Candau-Chacon, R, Chiu, H.J., Gehrke, B.J., et al. 2015. FDA approval: blinatumomab. *Clinical Cancer Research,* 21(18), 4035–4039.

Rajkumar, S.V. and Kumar, S. 2016. Multiple myeloma: diagnosis and treatment. *Mayo Clinic Proceedings,* 91(1), 101–119.

Rosenbaum, P.R. 2010. *Design of Observational Studies.* New York: Springer, vol. 10.

Rosenbaum, P.R., and Rubin, D.B. 1983. The central role of the propensity score in observational studies for causal effects. *Biometrika,* 70(1), 41–55.

Rosenbaum, P.R., and Rubin, D.B. 1984. Reducing bias in observational studies using subclassification on the propensity score. *Journal of the American Statistical Association,* 79(387), 516–524.

5

Bayesian Methods for Evaluating Drug Safety with Real-World Evidence

Binbing Yu

5.1 Introduction

Randomized controlled trials are the gold standard for establishing the efficacy of drugs [1]. However clinical trials for the purpose of registration are usually limited in size and duration and exclude high-risk populations. They tend to have limited statistical power to detect rare but potentially serious adverse events (SAEs) in real-world patients. The comprehensive review of design, analysis, and reporting issues for both clinical trials and observational studies in biopharmaceutical product development have been described in Jiang and Xia [2]. The typical challenges of the analysis of safety data from clinical trials include the lack of an evidentiary gold standard, a limited statistical power, the lack of adequate ascertainment of adverse events (AEs) and lack of generalizability, and external validity. Singh and Loke [1] discussed potential solutions to these challenges. Prieto-Merino et al. [3] discussed the use of pharmacovigilance system for detecting potential associations between drugs and AEs.

Regulatory agencies such as the U.S. Food and Drug Administration (FDA) and European Medicines Agency (EMA) have established elaborate and rigorous processes to demonstrate new drugs as safe and effective. Nonetheless, in recent years, several approved drugs have been withdrawn from the market because of serious and sometimes fatal side effects. For example, Rofecoxib (Vioxx) was voluntarily withdrawn from the market after a study showed that paitents taking the drug on a long-term basis have twice the risk of a heart attack compared with patients receiving placebo [4]. Bayesian methods have been used to evaluate drug safety issues [5]. The Bayesian methods are especially useful because of the high dimensionality of the data and for the ability of incorporating information from various sources [6].

In this chapter, we discuss the use of Bayesian methods to incorporate real-world evidence to assess the safety of drugs. We consider two case studies. The first one is using the Bayesian method to examine the impact of an unobserved confounder on the safety of spermicide. The second case is to assess whether a monoclonal antibody drug causes excess suicidal attempts for psoriasis patients.

5.2 Bayesian Sensitivity Analysis of an Unobserved Confounder

Unlike randomized clinical trials, investigators do not have control over the treatment assignment in observational studies. Without randomization, the treatment and control groups may have widely different distributions of relevant covariates. Even though bias due to observed confounders may be corrected using the regression analysis or matching techniques, the analyses may still be subject to potential bias arising from unobserved confounders. Sensitivity analysis is a technique for assessing whether the inference drawn from an observational study could be altered by a moderate "imbalance" between the distribution of the covariates in the treatment and control groups. There has been extensive research on how to perform sensitivity analysis for observational data in epidemiologic studies, for example, Cornfield et al. [7], Gastwirth [8], Rosenbaum [9], and others. Most of the literature considers models for the imbalance or association among the unobserved confounder, exposure, and response, and then recomputes the test statistics and p-values for a range of plausible association between the confounder and the exposure. If a moderate degree of confounding could change the estimate of the treatment effect, then the validity of the study findings is not robust.

By far, most methods of sensitivity analysis assume the parameters as fixed and vary the parameters within a plausible range. The Bayesian method treats the parameters as random and, thus, can incorporate sampling variability and historical information. McCandless et al. [10] considered Bayesian sensitivity analysis for the effect of an observed confounder when the exposure, response, and confounder are all binary variables. Here, we describe the Bayesian sensitivity analysis approach by using external real-world data. We apply the method to examine the robustness of an analysis concerning the possible effect of spermicide use on birth defects, that was cited in a legal decision [11].

5.2.1 Bayesian Sensitivity Analysis

Let X, Y, and U denote the exposure, response, and the unobserved confounder, respectively. Here we consider binary random variables for the triplets, where $Y = 1$ means event of interest and $Y = 0$ means no event. We assume that the probability of having an event follows a logistic model:

$$\text{logit}\{P_Y(Y = 1 \mid X, U)\} = \alpha + \beta X + \gamma U, \tag{5.1}$$

where the parameter β represents the effect of exposure on the probability of having an event. If the exposure variable is not a causal factor of the event, then $\beta = 0$. The Wald test can be used to examine whether the null hypothesis $H_0:\beta = 0$ is true. In general, also we can include the observed covariates Z in the regression analysis. For the simplicity of exposition, we omit the observed covariates Z in Eq. (5.1) and examine the potential impact of an unobserved confounder U. If the confounder U was observed, the parameter estimates would be obtained by the maximum likelihood method based on the logistic model (5.1).

In the actual analysis, the confounder U is not observed; hence, it is omitted from the analysis. The observed data with only X and Y can be presented as a 2×2 table. A reduced logistic model has to be used to estimate the association between X and Y,

$$\text{logit}\left\{P_Y^*\left(Y = 1 \mid X\right)\right\} = \alpha^* + \beta^* X. \tag{5.2}$$

For the unobserved confounder to explain the apparent association between X and Y if there is no such causal relationship, the variable U should be associated both X and Y as well. For a binary variable U, we also assume a logistic model for the association between U and X:

$$\text{logit}P_U\left(U = 1 \mid X\right) = \lambda + \delta X.$$

The quantity $\exp(\lambda)$ is the odds ratio of the association between U and X. Because the confounder U is not observed, it is treated as a missing value. Let $(y_i, x_i), i = 1, ..., n$ be the observed data. The likelihood function for the observed data is

$$L_1(\alpha, \beta, \gamma \mid X, Y) = \prod_{i=1}^{n} \int_u P_Y(Y = y_i \mid x_i, u) P_U(u \mid x_i) \, du.$$

Yu and Gastwirth [12] showed that if the unobserved variable U has a simultaneous relationship with the exposure X and response Y, the estimate of $\hat{\beta}^*$ from the reduced logistic model (5.2) is biased for the parameter β. Lin et al. [13] proposed a method for assessing the sensitivity of regression results to the unobserved confounders. As McCandless et al. [10] pointed out, in the situation where the model parameters are not identfiable, the Bayesian method with prior information may be used. They considered informative priors for all parameters γ, λ and δ, related to unobserved variable U. Here, we consider a slightly different scenario where the association of X and U can be obtained from historical data. Suppose that the association between X and U can be derived from a 2×2 table from historical data (Table 5.1). The likelihood function for the historical data in Table 5.2 is

$$L_2(\lambda, \delta \mid X, U) \propto \prod_{x=0}^{1} \prod_{u=0}^{1} P(U = u \mid X = x)^{m_{xj}}.$$

TABLE 5.1

Observed 2 × 2 Table for Exposure and Response

Exposure X	Response Y		Total
	0	1	
0	n_{00}	n_{01}	n_0
1	n_{10}	n_{11}	n_1

Let $\theta = (\alpha, \beta, \gamma, \lambda, \delta)$ be the set of parameters. The estimates of θ can be obtained by maximizing the joint likelihood $L(\theta) = L_1(\alpha, \beta, \gamma \mid X, Y)L_2(\lambda, \delta \mid X, U)$. Note that prior distributions for γ, λ, δ can be used to model the effect of unobserved confounder U. For example, if the parameter γ measures the log-odds ratio of U on response Y, one may assume an informative prior

$$\lambda \sim \text{Uniform}(L_\lambda, U_\lambda),$$

where L_λ and Y_λ are the lower and upper range of the possible values of λ based on expert opinion or meta-analysis. For a positive association, one may set the constraint that $\lambda > 0$. The priors for the parameters α and β that measure the effect of X on Y are assumed to be weakly or non-informative, e.g., $\beta \sim N(0,1000)$ to reflect a normal prior with large variance. The parameter estimates can be obtained using the Markov chain Monte Carlo (MCMC) method. The MCMC method has been implemented by the Bayesian inference package BUGS. The open-source application OpenBugs has been imbedded into the publicly available R package BRugs, which calls OpenBugs (https://www.mrc-bsu.cam.ac.uk/software/bugs/) [14].

5.2.2 Effect of Spermicide Use on Birth Defects

Motivated by a legal decision for *Wells vs. Ortho Pharmaceutical Corp.,* Gastwirth [15] examined the studies discussed in the decision to assess whether the critics, who claimed that the decision and its affirmation by the Court of Appeals showed that the legal system was unable to deal with scientific evidence, was justified. The decision found that limb defects of the babies were the result of the mothers' exposure to spermicide use after her

TABLE 5.2

Historical 2 × 2 Table for Exposure and Confounder

Exposure X	Confounder U		Total
	0	1	
0	m_{00}	m_{01}	m_0
1	m_{10}	m_{11}	m_1

TABLE 5.3

Cross-Tabulation of Limb Defect and
Spermicide Use After Last Menstrual Period

Limb Defect	Spermicide Use	
	No	Yes
No	2756	2208
Yes	75	75
Total	2831	2283

last menstrual period at the time the limb buds were formed. The court also found that there was sufficient evidence from two studies prior to the mothers' use of the drug that the defendant should have warned of an increased risk of limb defects. For example, Smith et al. [16] showed that spermicide was associated with limb defects with relative risk.

Here we examine the study that estimated the relationship between maternal spermicide use and congenital malformations [17]. Table 5.3 summarizes the number of limb defects (Y) by spermicide use (X) from the study. The estimated birth defect fractions are $p_0 = 2.65\%$ and $p_1 = 3.29\%$ for the spermicice non-users and users, respectively. The observed relative risk RR = p_1/p_0 = 1.24 with p-value 0.181. Therefore, the finding in [17] seems controversial and contradicts the belief that spermicide may lead to birth defects. However, Mills et al. [17] noted in the same study that spermicide users were significantly older, of higher parity and more educated than users of other birth control methods (all p-values < 0.0001), and they drank less alcohol and smoked fewer cigarettes ($p < 0.0001$).

It seems that smoking and drug use is an unobserved confounder for the association analysis in Table 5.3. In the same era, Polednak et al. [18] found that 31.4% of spermicide users past their last menstrual period smoked while 39.6% of non-users did. The 2×2 table for the spermicide use and smoking status are shown in Table 5.4. Smith et al. [16] also indicated that tranquilizer use was a risk factor with a similar relative risk. Later, Bracken and Holford [19] also found a relative risk of 3.7 for tranquilizer use and smoking for all birth defects. Is it possible that the non-significant association

TABLE 5.4

Cross-Tabulation of Smoking by Spermicide Use

Smoking	Spermicide Use	
	No	Yes
No	433	59
Yes	283	27
Total	716	86

TABLE 5.5

Estimates of the Parameters of the Association between Spermicide Use X, Smoking and Drug Use U and Birth Defect Y

Parameter	Estimate	Standard Error	p-Value	95% CI	
1. Association between X and Y from the Reduced Model					
α^*	−3.604	0.117	0.000	−3.833	−3.375
β^*	0.222	0.166	0.181	−0.103	0.547
2. Adjusted Parameters for Association between Y and X,U					
α	−5.548	1.188	0.000	−7.560	−3.669
β	0.419	0.235	0.074	−0.014	0.904
γ	2.700	1.391	0.052	0.182	4.893
3. Association Parameters between X and U					
λ	−0.427	0.076	0.000	−0.574	−0.278
δ	−0.378	0.248	0.129	−0.868	0.101

between spermicide use and limb defect at birth is due to the imbalance of smoking and drug use among the spermicide non-users and users?

We conducted a Bayesian sensitivity analysis to examine the effect of the unobserved variable of smoking and drug use. The smoking and drug use tend to increase the risk of birth defect. Therefore, we considered an informative prior $\gamma \sim$ Uniform (0,5). For the other parameters $\alpha, \beta, \lambda, \delta$, we use weekly informative prior $N(0, 1000)$. The final Bayesian estimates, which are the posterior means based on 10,000 MCMC samples after 5,000 burn-in samples, are summarized in Table 5.5. For comparison, the parameter estimates for α^* and β^* from the reduced logistic model (5.2) are shown in the top section. Without adjustment for the effect of unobserved variable U, the odds ratio of spermicide use on the birth defect is $\exp(0.222) = 1.249$ with a p-value 0.181. After adjusting for the unobserved confounder using the association data in Table 5.2, the odd ratio estimate of spermicide use is $\exp(0.419) = 1.520$ with a p-value 0.074. This indicates the the association between spermicide use and birth defect is borderline significant after adjustment of smoking and drug use. Therefore, the study results of non-signficant association between spermicide use and birth defect in Mills et al. [17] need further examinations before reaching a sound conclusion.

5.2.3 Concluding Remarks

Unobserved confounding is a common problem in observational studies. Various methods are available to control for observed confounders, either in the design of data collection by matching or exclusion, or in statistical analysis by multivariate regression or propensity score method [20]. Methods to quantify unobserved confounding can be categorized in those with and without prior knowledge of the effect estimate. Without prior knowledge of the effect estimate, the impact of unobserved confounding can be assessed using different types of sensitivity analysis. When prior knowledge is available, the size of unobserved confounding can be estimated directly by incorporation of prior knowledge. Bayesian sensitivity analysis is an appealing approach that incorporates prior knowledge and historical data to adjust the bias due to unobserved confounding.

5.3 Meta-Analysis of Drug Safety Data

Meta-analysis is a suite of statistical methods for systematic literature review with the goal to aggregate and contrast findings from several related studies [21–23]. Meta-analyses of clinical trial safety data have played important roles beyond regulatory submissions. During drug development, sponsors need to recognize safety signals early and adjust the development program accordinglys to facilitate the assessment of causality. Once a product is approved and sold on market, sponsors may conduct Phase IV clinical trial data to further understand existing or potential safety concerns in the real-world setting.

There is increasing demand by patients, healthcare providers, the biopharmaceutical industry, and society at large to have access to the total evidence on benefits and risks of drugs and biologics. This requires a comprehensive overview of all the available evidence whenever it is possible and sensible. For the evaluation of efficacy, the outcomes generally use the same or very similar pre-defined events for each of the trials to be included. Most regulatory guidance and many Cochrane Collaboration reviews have usually given more attention to assessment of benefits or efficacy. However, the meta-analysis of the safety of medicinal products have not been well investigated. This is in part due to the sparsity and unplanned nature of the safety data. Therefore, combining evidence on AEs or saftey issues is more challenging than combining evidence on pre-specified benefits. By combining safety data from different randomized controlled trials and observational studies and using proper statistical methods to evaluate this pooled information, we can provide a more precise measure of the safety of a product. This is especially true when it comes to events that may be uncommon or not specifically addressed by the primary outcome measures of a single clinical trial.

Here, we use the meta-analysis to estimate the rate of suicidal attempts for the patients in psoriasis from the population-based cohort studies. Based on the meta-analysis, we estimate the probability of observing a certain number of suicidal attempts in clinical trials given the background suicidal attempt rate.

5.3.1 Meta-Analysis for Evidence Synthesis

Here, we briefly describe the fixed and random effects for meta-analysis. Consider K studies and let y_i be the observed effect for the ith study, $i = 1, ..., K$. We assume that

$$y_i = \theta_i + \varepsilon_i, \tag{5.3}$$

where θ_i is the true effect, $\varepsilon_i \sim N(0, v_i)$ is the error term with variance v_i. The error variances are assumed to be known. Depending on the outcome measure used, a normalizing or transformation may be used to ensure that these assumptions are (approximately) true, i.e., logit transformation for rates and proportions.

Most meta-analyses are based on sets of studies that are not exactly identical in the methods and/or the characteristics of the patient population in the studies. Differences in the methods and patient characteristics may introduce variability among the true effects. One popular means for modeling the heterogeneity is to treat it as a random effect. This leads to the random-effects model, where the true effect

$$\theta_i = \mu + u_i, \tag{5.4}$$

where $u_i \sim N(0, \tau^2)$. The goal is then to estimate the average true effect μ and the heterogeneity τ^2 among the effects from different studies. When $\tau^2 = 0$, this reduces to a fixed-effect model. When using fixed-effects models, the goal is to make a conditional inference only about the K studies included in the meta-analysis [24]. If weighted least squares is used to fit the model, then the estimate of average effect from the fixed-effects model is

$$\bar{\theta} = \sum_i w_i \theta / \sum_i w_i, \tag{5.5}$$

where the weights are typically set equal to $w_i = 1 / v_i$.

The random-effects meta-analytic model is essentially a special case of the linear mixed-effects model. Therefore, the parameter estimates can be obtained from the linear mixed-effects model estimation procedure. Once the parameter estimates have been obtained, Wald-type tests and confidence intervals (CIs) then can be easily obtained for the parameters μ and τ^2. Estimation of the meta-analytic models have been implemented in various R packages, including `metafor` [25] and `meta` [26].

5.3.2 Suicidal Risk of Brodalumab

Psoriasis is a chronic autoimmune disease in which the growth cycle of skin cells is accelerated. Genetic and environmental factors induce immune responses mediated by several cytokines and chemokines, including inter-leukin-17 (IL-17) [27, 28]. IL-17 is a cytokine that controls cells and activates inflammation. For healthy individuals without psoriasis, these molecules stimulate the body's immune system into action only when there is a cut or a scrape, sending cells to the surface to fight infection and heal a wound. Psoriasis patients have 30 times more IL-17 than healthy people. Research has shown that stopping IL-17, or reducing it, may help clear psoriasis.

Brodalumab, secukinumab, and ixekizumab all work by interfering with the IL-17 pathway. Secukinumab and ixekizumab target IL-17, whereas broda-lumab targets a specific receptor that binds to the IL-17 cytokine. Brodalumab is a novel human monoclonal antibody that binds to the IL-17 receptor and inhibits inflammatory signaling by blocking the binding of several types of IL-17 to the receptor. The safety and efficacy of two doses of brodalumab com-pared with placebo and ustekinumab (Stelara) were assessed in two Phase 3 multi-arm pivotal trials, i.e., AMAGINE-2 and AMAGINE-3, in patients with moderate-to-severe plaque psoriasis. Patients treated with brodalumab treat-ment had significant clinical improvement [29]. Specifically, brodalumab was superior to ustekinumab on the primary endpoint of achieving total clearance of skin disease, as measured by the patients achieving completely clear skin (PASI100). The week 12 PASI100 response rates with 210 mg of brodalumab were significantly higher than with ustekinumab (44% vs. 22% [AMAGINE-2] and 37% vs. 19% [AMAGINE-3], p-value < 0.001). The PASI 100 response rates among the 140-mg brodalumab group also were higher than those among the ustekinumab. Although brodalumab was highly effective and had a compa-rable safety profile in many SAEs and AEs, there were events of suicidal ten-dencies and actual suicides that occurred in the two Phase 3 trials. The FDA approved brodalumab (Siliq) to treat adults with moderate-to-severe plaque psoriasis, however, with a black box warning that "suicidal ideation and behaviour, including completed suicides, have occurred in patients treated with Siliq during clinical trial." This warning pose a big challenge to the sponsor who tried to compete against other IL-17 inhibitors.

Even though suicidal ideation is a serious safety issue, it is quite a rare event. People may question: "Is the association between suicide risk and brodalumab use real, bad luck. or simply a false alarm?" A real connection implies a causal relationship that leads to higher suicide tendency. This requires the estab-lishment of a scientific mechanism targeting the IL-17 receptor that, indeed, causes suicide tendencies. Bad luck suggests a statistical fluke in the data, potentially caused by the generally higher background prevalence of suicide risk in the moderate-to-severe psoriasis patient population or other uncon-trolled or unaccounted confounding factors. If the basis of brodalumab caus-ing suicide can be ruled out both scientifically and statistically, the observed suicidal risk in the brodalumab might be simply a false alarm.

The goals of the analysis are (1) to investigate whether the suicidal risk for patients in the brodalumab treatment group is statistically higher than those for the untreated psoriasis patients and the patients treated with secukinumab or ixekizumab and (2) whether an unobserved confounder or latent risk factors can explain the higher suicidal risk in AMAGINE-2 and AMAGINE-3 trials. We reanalyzed the public-available safety data from the two Phase 3 pivotal trials for brodalumab. Particularly, we focus on the effect of suicide risk, because the risks of other SAEs and AEs are comparable to the placebo groups.

5.3.3 Statistical Evaluation of Suicidal Risk

A PubMed and EMBASE database search was conducted with "suicide AND psoriasis" as search terms on March 15, 2016. The limit for the PubMed search was English in the title/abstract field. Limits for the EMBASE search were articles published after 2006. The population-based cohort studies of psoriasis were selected to determine the suicidal risk of the general psoriasis patient population. The incidence rates of suicidality from the selected population-based cohort/registry study are shown in Table 5.6. A meta-analysis was conducted to calculate the overall incidence rate of suicidality in the general psoriasis patient population. The meta-analysis using the random-effects model shows that the overall incidence rate is 0.57 per 1,000 person-year with 95% CI (0.25, 0.84) per 1,000 person-years.

The safety data for the clinical trials for brodalumab, secukinumab, and ixekizumab were obtained from published articles or conference presentations [29, 33–34]. The number of suicide attempts or deaths and number of subjects and person-years at risk are shown in Table 5.7. Based on data from Tables 5.6 and 5.7, we can examine whether the suicidal risk in the treatment group in the clinical trials, particularly whether the suicidal risk in the AMAGINE-2 and AMAGINE-3 trials for brodalumab, are significantly higher than that for the general psoriasis paitient population.

TABLE 5.6

Incidence Rates of Suicidal Attempt from the Population-Based Cohort or Registry Studies

Reference	Patient	Number of Subjects	Number of Cases	Incidence Rate per 1,000 Person-years
Abuabara et al. (2010) [30]	Severe psoriasis	3,603	1	0.2
Kurd et al. (2010)	Mild psoriasis	146,042	Not reported	0.93
	Severe psoriasis	3,956	Not reported	0.92
Singhal et al. (2014) [31]	Psoriasis	119,304	1,141	0.74
Svedbom, et al. (2015) [32]	Mild psoriasis	34,355	27	0.17
	Severe psoriasis	4,719	3	0.19

TABLE 5.7

Number of Cases, Subjects, and Exposure for Several Phase 2, 3 Trials for Brodalumab, Secukinmab, and Ixekizumab

Drug	Clinical Trial	Duration	Dose	Number of Subjects	Exposure	Number of Suicides
Brodalumab	AMAGINE-2 & AMAGINE-3	54+ weeks	210 mg Q2W	975	781.2	2
		12 weeks	210 mg Q2W	1,234	284.8	1
Secukinumab	Pooled 7 clinical trials	Vary	≥ 1 dose	39,28	3225.0	2
Ixekizumab	UNCOVER-2 and UNCOVER-3	12 weeks	Q2W	7,29	168.2	1
		12 weeks	Q4W	734	169.4	1

In Table 5.7, the risk of suicidal attempts at week 12 were comparable for the AMAGINE-2 and AMAGINE-3 210-mg Q2W dose group and the UNCOVER-2 and UNCOVER-3 trials. Actually, the exposure-adjusted incidence rate of suicidal attempt in the AMAGINE-2 and AMAGINE-3 trials was lower than that in the UNCOVER-2 and UNCOVER-3 trials at week 12. Most of the suicidal attempts occurred in the 210-mg Q2W group with constant dose. One patient committed three suicidal attempts before week 52, and one additional suicide occurred after week 52 during the open-label extension in the AMAGINE-2 study [29]. The three suicidal attempts are strongly correlated. In the analysis, we count the three attempts as one incidence case. We can assess the probability of observing such numbers of suicidal cases given the incidence rates from the general patient population. We estimate the probability from the Bayesian perspective. Based on the meta-analysis for the suicidal incidence from population-based cohorts in Table 5.6, the logit of the incidence rate λ is distributed as

$$\text{logit}(\lambda) \sim N\left(\mu_\lambda, \sigma_\lambda\right) \tag{5.6}$$

with $\mu_\lambda = 0.27$ and $\sigma_\lambda = 0.69$. The null hypothesis to be tested is that H_0: the suicidal risk in the brodalumab clinical trials is similar to that of the general psoriasis patients. In the clinical trials, the number of suicidal attempt cases Y follows a Poisson distribution

$$Y \sim \text{Poisson}(n\lambda), \tag{5.7}$$

where n is the person-years of exposure to the treatment and λ is the incidence rate of suicidal attempt for the psoriasis patients. If the null hypothesis

TABLE 5.8

Probability of Observing the Number of Suicide Cases in the AMAGINE-2 and AMAGINE-3 Trials for Brodalumab

Duration	Number of Subjects	Exposure	Number of suicides (y)	$P(Y \geq y)$
54+ weeks	975	781.2	2	0.067
12 weeks	1,234	284.8	1	0.138

is true, the probability of observing y number of suicidal attempts in the brodalumab clinical trial is

$$P(Y \geq y) = \int P(Y \geq y \mid n\lambda) f(\lambda) d\lambda = \sum_{k \geq y} \int \frac{(n\lambda)^k e^{-n\lambda}}{k!} f(\lambda) d\lambda, \qquad (5.8)$$

where $f(\lambda)$ is the density function of the background suicidal incidence rates based on Eq. (5.6).

Based on the background suicidal incidence rate estimated from the meta-analysis, the probabilities of observing a certain number of suicidal cases for the two clinical trials for brodalumab are shown in Table 5.8. At the study duration of 54+ weeks, there are 975 patients who receive a 210-mg constant dose Q2W and the total exposure time is 781.2 person-year; the posterior mean probability of observing two suicidal subjects or more is $P(Y \geq 2) = 0.067$. The corresponding probability for the one case at week 12 is 0.138. Therefore, given the higher background risk of suicidal attempts among the psoriasis patients, it is possible that even though the use of brodalumab did not cause additional risk of suicide, we may still observe two or more suicidal attempts in the AMAGINE-2 and AMAGINE-3. In addition, multiple AEs are monitored in the safety analysis; the chance of an AE being statistically significant is even higher due to multiple testing. Note that the one subject at week 54 attempted suicide three times. If we count the three suicidal attempts as independent, we may observe four suicidal attempts by week 54. The probability of observing four or more cases is 0.0013. This may indicate a possibility of brodalumab causing suicide. However, this probability estimate is extremely conservative as the multiple suicidal attempts for the same individual are strongly correlated.

Furthermore, there may be some other causal factors related to the suicidal cases for brodalumab. First, antidepressant use might be a confounder that is associated with suicidal risk. Psoriasis patients are increasingly exposed to antidepressant drugs [35], and the use of antidepressants has been linked to suicidality and aggression [36]. Since May 2014, AMAGINE-2 and AMAGINE-3 started to collect information about the depression scale, but without further information, we cannot run a thorough analysis. In an earlier PLATO trial for Brilinta for cardiovascular diseases, the excessive use of aspirin has been shown to explain the regional difference of relative risk of cardiovascular death [37]. As a confounder, the excess use of antidepressants may explain the difference of suicidal attempts between the brodalumab and placebo groups. In the absence of a control group in the open-label period, it is possible that the additional one reported suicide may be caused by another crisis not related to drug use. For example, worsening symptoms or recent economic crisis in the United States were associated with an increase in the suicidal rate [38].

5.3.4 Concluding Remarks

Although there are many systemic agents approved for the treatment of psoriasis, getting patients clear of their psoriasis is still a hurdle. Secukinumab (Cosentyx), an inhibitor of IL-17, was approved for the treatment of moderate-to-severe psoriasis in 2015. Two other inhibitors of IL-17, brodalumab and ixekizumab, also are approved by the FDA for treatment of psoriasis. There has been no suicidality signal with secukinumab, nor with ixekizumab. Furthermore, antagonism of cytokine activity, and particularly of cytokines IL-6, IL-17, and IL-23, has not been associated with neurological symptoms. For example, the anti–IL-6 receptor antibody tocilizumab has shown a positive impact in rheumatoid arthritis patients' quality-of-life scoring, which includes fatigue, anxiety, depression, and a number of other factors. More to the point, the anti–IL-17 antibody secukinumab, which targets the IL-17 ligand (rather than the receptor), has not shown a link to suicide. Given the statistical analysis of real-world evidence, people may cast doubt on the claim that brodalumab increases the risk of suicide. Clearly more data are needed, and it would not be surprising if the FDA began a drug class review if the data in the brodalumab trials warranted it. They could cast quite a wide net given the complexity of this pathway, which overlaps with IL-6, IL-12, and IL-23.

5.4 Summary

Increasing scientific, regulatory, and public scrutiny focuses on the obligation of the medical community, pharmaceutical industry, and health authorities to ensure that marketed drugs have acceptable benefit-risk profiles. Randomized control trials have long been considered the cornerstone of evidence-based medicine. They are, however, not always feasible due to financial, ethical, and practical constraints, and are criticized for the lack of external validity. Real-world data may provide a useful alternative for assessing the safety of drugs and biologics. A key challenge in observational studies is confounding. Although extensive research has been conducted on the estimation of efficacy to account for confounding, there is limited literature on the assessment of drug safety in the presence of confounding.

We consider two case studies that use the Bayesian method to utilize real-world data to assess the safety of drugs. The method is easy to implement and may be a promising approach for drug safety assessment [39]. However, there also are many challenges in the assessment of drug safety using real-world data. The data quality and patient population from heterogeneous sources should be thoroughly examined to ensure the findings are robust and reliable.

References

1. Singh, S. and Loke, Y.K. 2012. Drug safety assessment in clinical trials: methodological challenges and opportunities. *Trials*, 13, 138.
2. Jiang, Q. and Xia, H.A. 2014. *Quantitative Evaluation of Safety in Drug Development: Design, Analysis and Reporting*, Bio-Statistics Series, London: Taylor & Francis.
3. Prieto-Merino, D., Quartey, G., Wang, J., and Kim, J. 2011. Why a Bayesian approach to safety analysis in pharmacovigilance is important. *Pharmaceutical Statistics*, 10(6), 554–559.
4. Sibbald, B. 2004. Rofecoxib (Vioxx) voluntarily withdrawn from market. *Canadian Medical Association Journal*, 171(9), 1027–1028.
5. Xia, H.A., Ma, H., and Carlin, B.P. 2011. Bayesian hierarchical modeling for detecting safety signals in clinical trials. *Journal of Bio-Pharmaceutical Statistics*, 21(5), 1006–1029.
6. Madigan, D., Ryan, P., Simpson, S., and Zorych, I. 2010. Bayesian methods in pharmacovigilance. *Bayesian Statistics*, 9, 421–438.
7. Cornfield, J., Haenszel, W., Hammond, E.C., Lilienfeld, A.M., Shimkin, M.B., and Wynder, E.L. 1959. Smoking and lung cancer: recent evidence and a discussion of some questions. *Journal of the National Cancer Institute*, 22(1), 173–203.
8. Gastwirth, J.L. 1988. *Statistical Reasoning in Law and Public Policy*. Boston, MA: Academic Press.
9. Rosenbaum, P.R. 2002. Observational studies. *Observational Studies*, Springer Science & Business Media, New York.
10. McCandless, L.C., Gustafson, P., and Levy, A. 2007. Bayesian sensitivity analysis for unmeasured confounding in observational studies. *Statistics in Medicine*, 26(11), 2331–2347.
11. Gastwirth, J.L. and Greenhouse, S.W. 1995. Biostatistical concepts and methods in the legal setting. *Statistics in Medicine*, 14(15), 1641–1653.
12. Yu, B. and Gastwirth, J. L. 2003. The use of the reverse cornfield inequality to assess the sensitivity of a nonsignificant association to an omitted variable. *Statistics in Medicine*, 22(21), 3383–3401.
13. Lin, D. Y., Psaty, B. M., and Kronmal, R. A. 1998. Assessing the sensitivity of regression results to unmeasured confounders in observational studies. *Biometrics*, 54(3), 948.
14. Thomas, A., O'Hara, B., Ligges, U., and Sturtz, S. 2006. Making BUGS open. *R News*, 6(1), 12–17.
15. Gastwirth, J.L. 2003. The need for careful evaluation of epidemiological evidence in product liability cases: a reexamination of Wells v. Ortho and Key Pharmaceuticals. *Law, Probability and Risk*, 2(3), 151–189.

16. Smith, E.S.O., Dafoe, C.S., Miller, J.R., and Banister, P. 1977. An epidemiological study of congenital reduction deformities of the limbs. *British Journal of Preventive and Social Medicine*, 31(1), 39–41.

17. Mills, J.L., Harley, E.E., Reed, G.F., and Berendes, H.W. 1982. Are spermicides teratogenic? *JAMA*, 248(17), 2148–2151.

18. Polednak, A.P., Janerich, D.T., and Glebatis, D.M. 1982. Birth weight and birth defects in relation to maternal spermicide use. *Teratology*, 26(1), 27–38.

19. Bracken, M.B. and Holford, T.R. 1981. Exposure to prescribed drugs in pregnancy and association with congenital malformations. *Obstetrics and Gynecology*, 58(3), 336–344.

20. Groenwold, R.H.H., Hak, E., and Hoes, A.W. 2009. Quantitative assessment of unobserved confounding is mandatory in nonrandomized intervention studies. *Journal of Clinical Epidemiology*, 62(1), 22–28.

21. Hedges, L.V. and Olkin, I. 1985. *Statistical Methods for Meta-Analysis*. San Diego, CA: Academic Press.

22. Van Houwelingen, H.C., Arends, L.R., and Stijnen, T. 2002. Advanced methods in meta-analysis: multivariate approach and meta-regression. *Statistics in Medicine*, 21(4), 589–624.

23. Raudenbush, S. W. 2009. Analyzing effect sizes: random-effects models. In *The Handbook of Research Synthesis and Meta-Analysis*, New York: Russell Sage Foundation, 295–315.

24. Hedges, L.V. and Vevea, J.L. 1998. Fixed- and random-effects models in meta-analysis. *Psychological Methods*, 3(4), 486–504.

25. Viechtbauer, W. 2010. Conducting meta-analyses in R with the metafor. *Journal of Statistical Software*, 36(3), 1–48.

26. Schwarzer, G. and Schwarzer, M.G. 2012. Package meta. *The R Foundation for Statistical Computing*, 9.

27. Chiricozzi, A. and Krueger, J.G. 2013. Il-17 targeted therapies for psoriasis. *Expert Opinion on Investigational Drugs*, 22(8), 993–1005.

28. Gooderham, M., Posso-De Los Rios, C.J., Rubio-Gomez, G.A., and Papp, K. 2015. Interleukin-17 (il-17) inhibitors in the treatment of plaque psoriasis: a review. *Skin Therapy Letters*, 20(1), 1–5.

29. Lebwohl, M., Strober, B., Menter, A., Gordon, K., Weglowska, J., Puig, L., Papp, K., Spelman, L., Toth, D., Kerdel, F., et al. 2015. Phase 3 studies comparing brodalumab with ustekinumab in psoriasis. *New England Journal of Medicine*, 373(14), 1318–1328.

30. Abuabara, K., Azfar, R.S., Shin, D.B., Neimann, A.L., Troxel, A.B. and Gelfand, J.M., 2010. Cause-specific mortality in patients with severe psoriasis: a population-based cohort study in the UK. *British Journal of Dermatology*, 163(3), 586–592.

31. Singhal, A., Ross, J., Seminog, O., Hawton, K. and Goldacre, M.J., 2014. Risk of self-harm and suicide in people with specific psychiatric and physical disorders: comparisons between disorders using English national record linkage. *Journal of the Royal Society of Medicine*, 107(5), 194–204.

32. Svedbom, A., Dalen, J., Mamolo, C., Cappelleri, J.C., Mallbris, L., Petersson, I.F. and Ståhle, M., 2015. Increased cause-specific mortality in patients with mild and severe psoriasis: a population-based Swedish register study. *Acta dermato-venereologica*, 95(7), 809–815.

33. Mease, P., McInnes, I.B., Richards, H., Pricop, L., Widmer, A., and Mpofu, S. 2015. Sat0579 secukinumab safety and tolerability in patients with active psoriatic

arthritis: Pooled safety analysis of two phase 3, randomized, controlled trials (future 1 and future 2). *Annals of the Rheumatic Diseases,* 74(Suppl 2), 870.3–871.

34. Griffiths, C.E.M., Reich, K., Lebwohl, M., van de Kerkhof, P.C., Menter, A., Cameron, G.S., Erickson, J., Zhang, L., Secrest, R.J., et al. 2015. Comparison of ixekizumab with etanercept or placebo in moderate-to-severe psoriasis (uncover-2 and uncover-3): results from two phase 3 randomised trials. *Lancet,* 386(9993), 541–551.

35. Dowlatshahi, E.A., Wakkee, M., Herings, R., Hollestein, L.M, and Nijsten, T. 2013. Increased antidepressant drug exposure in psoriasis patients: a longitudinal population-based cohort study. *Acta Dermato-Venereologica,* 93(5), 544–550.

36. Sharma, T., Guski, L.S., Freund, N., and Gøtzsche, P.C. 2016. Suicidality and aggression during antidepressant treatment: systematic review and meta-analyses based on clinical study reports. *BMJ,* 352, i65.

37. Carroll, K.J. and Fleming, T.R. 2013. Statistical evaluation and analysis of regional interactions: the Plato trial case study. *Statistics in Bio-Pharmaceutical Research,* 5(2), 91–101.

38. Danesh, M.J. and Kimball, A.B. 2016. Brodalumab and suicidal ideation in the context of a recent economic crisis in the united states. *Journal of the American Academy of Dermatology,* 74(1), 190–192.

39. Ohlssen, D., Price, K.L., Xia, H.A., Hong, H., Kerman, J., Fu, H., Quartey, G., Heilmann, C.R., Ma, H., and Carlin, B.P. 2013. Guidance on the implementation and reporting of a drug safety Bayesian network meta-analysis. *Pharmaceutical Statistics,* 13(1), 55–70.

6

Real-World Evidence for Coverage and Payment Decisions

Saurabh Aggarwal, Hui Huang, Ozlem Topaloglu, Ross Selby
Hui Huang, Saurabh (Rob) Aggarwal

6.1 Introduction

The rise in healthcare spending is posing a challenge for payers and policy makers to manage budgets across several markets[1]. As choices increase, payers and other stakeholders are demanding a demonstration of value of medical products to justify payment.

The recent high price of breakthrough medical treatments such as gene therapies (priced at $500,0000–$2,000,000 per treatment) has reignited the debate on the value of medical products[2-4]. The large pipeline of novel therapies has raised the issue of affordability, in terms of providing access to new treatment, while continuing to provide coverage of treatments for larger populations[2,5]. There is also a gap in efficacy and effectiveness, especially for orphan medical products that are approved by regulatory agencies based on short-term, surrogate endpoints and/or single-arm studies in special populations[6]. Due to these cost pressures and gap in efficacy effectiveness, stakeholders are increasingly demanding additional proof of value of medical treatments beyond the typical pivotal trials for regulatory approval. Real-world evidence (RWE) offers an opportunity to demonstrate effectiveness and safety in populations that are relevant to payers.

6.2 Defining Value

There has been an ongoing effort by several stakeholders to use a "value"-based metric for making coverage and payment decisions[1,7,8]. However, there is no clear consensus for the definition of value and the process for value assessment[9]. Various stakeholders such as payers, health technology assessment (HTA) agencies, and medical societies have taken and/or proposed different methods for value assessment. There are multiple value frameworks that currently exist (Table 6.1).

The International Society for Pharmacoeconomics & Outcomes Research (ISPOR) task force raised concerns regarding these value frameworks saying some of these pose greater threats to their face validity and utility compared with others[10]. According to the ISPOR task force, the most significant

TABLE 6.1

Value Frameworks Overview

Framework	Brief Description	Website
ICER Value Framework	Based on two general concepts: "long-term value for money" and "short-term affordability." Long-term value for money is measured based on incremental cost per quality adjusted life years (QALYs). Short-term affordability is based on total costs (medical and product related) for the entire healthcare system over a time period of 5 years.	https://icer-review.org/material/2020-value-assessment-framework-final-framework/
NCCN Evidence Blocks™	National Comprehensive Cancer Network (NCCN) panel members score five measures on a scale of 1 to 5. The five measures are Efficacy of Regimen/Agent, Safety of Regimen/Agent, Quality of Evidence, Consistency of Evidence, and Affordability of Regimen/Agent.	https://www.nccn.org/evidenceblocks/
American Society of Clinical Oncology (ASCO) Net Health Benefit Score	Estimates a "Net Health Benefit score," derived from the key efficacy elements of overall survival (OS), progression-free survival (PFS), response rate (RR), symptom palliation, time off treatment, and quality of life (QoL), along with the comparative toxicity of the regimen.	https://ascopubs.org/doi/full/10.1200/JCO.2016.68.2518
European Society for Medical Oncology Magnitude of Clinical Benefit Scale (ESMO-MCBS)	Assessment depends on whether the treatment is curative or non-curative. Score is based on clinical, QoL and safety evidence (version 1.1).	https://www.esmo.org/Guidelines/ESMO-MCBS/Articles/ESMO-Magnitude-of-Clinical-Benefit-Scale-version-1.1
DrugAbacus	Interactive cancer drug pricing tool based on (1) price for a year of life, (2) toxicity, (3) novelty, (4) rare disease setting, (5) burden of disease, (6) cost of development, (7) prognosis, and (8) unmet need.	https://drugpricinglab.org/tools/drug-abacus/

limitations include lack of clear perspective (e.g., patient vs. health plan) and poor transparency in accounting for costs and benefits[10].

6.3 Contracting Trends/Value-Based Agreements

During the past few years, many different types of value-based agreements have been made between payers and product manufacturers. These agreements provide payment or rebate based on real-world outcomes of the product. Different terms have been used for value-based agreements, such as "outcomes-based contracts (OBC)," "value-based pricing," "performance-based contracts," "value-based contracts," "risk-sharing agreements," "coverage with evidence development," and "managed entry schemes"[8,11,12].

6.3.1 Outcomes-Based Contracts

An OBC ties payment to the real-world outcomes in the payer's population[13]. The OBCs have been implemented in some European markets such as Italy, Sweden, the United Kingdom, and Germany. In the United States, the number of OBCs have been increasing. Although some countries have established mechanisms for generating and reporting RWE (e.g., Italy and Sweden), the process is still uncertain in other countries[14]. In a survey conducted by the Academy of Managed Care Pharmacy (AMCP), the majority of US payers and manufacturers reported having an interest in OBCs. However, until recently, actual use of such contracts has been limited due to challenges in collecting real-world outcomes[13,15]. In the future, as operational challenges are mitigated with use of electronic health records and partnerships with payers and integrated healthcare systems, the OBCs could emerge as an effective pathway to manage access using real-world outcomes.

6.3.2 Financial-Based Agreements

In financial-based agreements the payment is based on financial considerations and is not related to clinical performance. Examples include price-volume agreements, cost capitation, and free product for a certain number of cycles of treatment. For example, in South Korea if a pharmaceutical product's use was increased by 30–60%, it would lead to a 10% reduction in price[16]. Another example is the new "Netflix model" of fixed/subscription fee paid by the payer for unlimited access to treatment. In 2019, Louisiana and Washington states announced plans to reimburse for hepatitis C treatment in Medicaid through supplemental rebate agreements using a Netflix-style subscription model[17,18].

6.3.3 Alternative/Innovative Payment Models

In recent years, some innovative payment models have been proposed that amortize the cost of treatment over multiple years. Amortization can be potentially combined with an outcomes-based agreement in the form of milestone-based payments[19]. In 2018, AveXis and Novartis announced that cost of Zolgensma (gene therapy for treatment of spinal muscular atrophy) will be annualized to $425,000 per year for 5 years, creating 5-year outcomes-based agreements and novel pay-over-time options[20].

6.4 Importance of RWE for Demonstrating Value

6.4.1 RWE for Product Effectiveness

More payers and other stakeholders are increasingly demanding evidence for a product's effectiveness in their coverage populations. Studies to generate this evidence can be conducted either by the product manufacturer, or payer, or as a joint collaboration from multiple stakeholders. A real-world study by Takeda Pharmaceuticals in Germany and the United Kingdom showed that brentuximab vedotin is effective in autologous stem cell transplant (ASCT)-ineligible patients with relapsed/refractory Hodgkin lymphoma (rrHL)[21]. Kaiser Permanente Northern California has a viral hepatitis registry that includes administrative and clinical data for all patients with chronic hepatitis C[22]. Recently, many new joint collaborations between a product manufacturer and a payer/HTA were announced to align reimbursement to real-world outcomes in the payer/HTA's target population. For example, Merck and United Health's Optum have an initiative that involves the use of real-world data to co-develop and test advanced predictive models and co-design an outcome-based risk sharing agreement to reduce clinical and financial uncertainty[23].

6.4.2 RWE for Product Safety

Safety evidence is required as part of the regulatory approval process. However, for some products and in some disease settings, payers also are interested in other safety outcomes (e.g., risks of malignancies, cardiovascular events) and long-term assessment of risk in a real-world setting. In a survey of payers, the product safety was mentioned as one of the reasons for leveraging RWE[24]. A recent study by Kaiser Permanente examined the risk for malignancy and mortality in 8,219 human immunodeficiency virus (HIV)-infected raltegravir-treated patients. The study demonstrated how payers can conduct observational studies using their database to assess real-world safety risks[25].

6.4.3 RWE for HEOR Outcomes

In addition to safety and efficacy, RWE also can be leveraged to generate evidence for payers/HTAs for health economics and outcomes research (HEOR) outcomes such as quality of life, patient-reported outcomes (PROs), work productivity, adherence, and cost-effectiveness in a real-world setting. For example, adherence is a major concern for payers, as non-compliance leads to poor clinical outcomes and potentially higher resource use and therefore a higher economic burden. In a study using data from Humana, schizophrenia patients who were adherent had lower hospitalizations and medical costs[26].

6.4.4 RWE for Burden of Disease

Another aspect of the product value is the burden-of-illness value proposition. If stakeholders are not aware of the seriousness of the disease and unmet need, it is likely they will not value the product. RWE from previous and new studies can be used to build awareness about the burden of illness of a disease[27]. For example, for influenza, a large multicenter observational study in Canada showed that the average length of hospital stay was 10.8 days, general ward stays were 9.4 days, and intensive care unit stays were 9.8 days[28]. Such studies are useful to educate payers about the high burden of the disease. In a recent assessment by the Institute for Clinical and Economic Review (ICER), the Familial Amyloidotic Polyneuropathy World Transplant Registry data were used to show the burden of liver transplantation in patients with hereditary transthyretin amyloidosis[29].

6.5 Use of RWE by Payers and Health Technology Assessment Agencies

6.5.1 Targeted Literature Review

A targeted review of the literature was conducted to identify publications on trends, case studies, and guidance from 2017–2019 for use of RWE by payers and HTAs. PubMed and Embase databases were searched and screened to select the latest full-text publications and conference abstracts.

6.5.2 Findings from the Review of Studies on Trends in Use of RWE by Payers

The targeted review identified seven studies that analyzed the use of RWE in the HTA process. The HTAs covered included ICER (United States), National Institute for Health and Care Excellence (NICE; England, Wales),

Scottish Medicines Consortium (SMC; Scotland), Haute Autorité de Santé (HAS; France), Institute for Quality and Efficacy in Healthcare (IQWIG; Germany), Pan-Canadian Oncology Drug Review (pCODR; Canada), Pharmaceutical Benefits Advisory Committee (PBAC; Australia), Agency for Health Technology Assessment and Tariff Systems (AOTMiT; Poland), and Zorginstituut Nederland (ZIN; the Netherlands). Overall, more than half of the HTA reports included RWE (range 45–100%; Table 6.2). The most common uses of RWE were for epidemiology, clinical effectiveness, and cost-effectiveness.

In a review of 52 HTA reports on melanoma by 5 HTA agencies, RWE was used in 88% of the reports for cost-effectiveness analyses and 54% for relative effectiveness[30]. However, the use of RWE varies by HTA agency. For example, for melanoma, 10 of 10 assessments by NICE used RWE for effectiveness, whereas SMC used it only for 3 of 10 assessments. IQWIG, ZIN, and HAS assessments had used RWE mainly for epidemiology[30]. For cost-effectiveness analyses, the use of RWE was more than 75% by NICE, SMC, and ZIN[30].

In the United States, ICER was found to use RWE for effectiveness in 46% of the reports[31]. Additionally, in systematic literature reviews (SLRs) conducted as part of ICER's assessment, 58% of the SLRs included RWE[31].

Similarly, the use of RWE was more than 50% in 16 HTA reports for the non-small cell lung cancer (NSCLC) published by NICE, pCODR, PBAC, and HAS[32]. Although 10 of 13 appraisals from NICE, 6 of 9 of PBAC, and 6 of 10 of pCODR included RWE, none of the 7 reports by HAS had used RWE[32]. This is likely due to NICE's requirement for generating RWE for coverage under the Cancer Drug Fund (CDF). In Australia, manufacturers are expected to collect RWE for overall survival using registry-based studies[32].

A review of assessments of Poland's AOTMiT showed that on average RWE was considered in 45% of the reports, with mostly observational studies.

A recent review of NICE's 2016–2017 assessments found 19 reports in which NICE requested, considered, or accepted the use of RWE. In these reports, RWE was mentioned 10 times for cost-effectiveness, 6 for clinical effectiveness, 5 for clinical management, 3 for dosage, 4 for overall survival extrapolation, and 2 for utility score[33]. In a review of 84 pCODR reports on cancer drugs, almost half of them included recommendations to generate RWE to address data gaps[34].

RWE is especially useful for rare diseases, where small populations make it challenging to conduct large population studies or randomized pivotal trials. In a review of NICE's assessments for products indicated for ultra-orphan diseases [covered under the Highly Specialized Technology (HST) program] all 7 of 7 (100%) appraisals were found to use RWE for effectiveness, safety, dosing trends, or natural history of the disease[27].

TABLE 6.2

Studies on Use of RWE by HTAs

Author Year	Payer/HTA	Study Method	Key Finding
Drane et al. 2019[31]	ICER (US)	Review of 26 assessment reports	15 of 26 (58%) assessments included RWE in the SLR. 12 of 26 (46%) used RWE for demonstrating comparative clinical effectiveness.
Makady et al. 2018[30]	NICE (UK), SMC (Scotland), HAS (France), IQWIG (Germany), ZIN (the Netherlands)	Review of 52 HTA reports on melanoma published between January 1, 2011 and December 31, 2016	RWE was included in 28 of the 52 reports (54%), mainly to estimate melanoma prevalence, and in 22 of 25 (88%) CEAs, mainly to extrapolate long-term effectiveness and/or identify drug-related costs.
Ng et al. 2018[32]	NICE (UK), HAS (France), pCODR (Canada), and PBAC (Australia)	16 NSCLC HTA reports	RWE was submitted in 56% of the appraisals, specifically 10/13 of NICE appraisals, 6/9 of PBAC, 6/10 of pCODR, and 0/7 of HAS.
Wilk et al. 2017[35]	AOTMiT (Poland)	Review of 58 assessments	The average proportion of RWE in evidence considered was 45%.
Aggarwal et al. 2018[33]	NICE (UK)	Review of 19 HTA reports (2016–2017)	19 HTA reports were found for which NICE requested, considered, or accepted use of RWE. There were 30 different references for RWE in the 19 reports: 10 for cost-effectiveness, 6 for clinical effectiveness, 5 for clinical management, 3 for dosage, 4 for overall survival extrapolation, and 2 for utility scores.
Han et al. 2018[34]	pCODR (Canada)	Review of 84 reports (January 2012 to May 2017)	41 of 84 (48%) included the next step of generating RWE to address data gaps.
Aggarwal and Topaloglu 2019[27]	NICE (UK)	Review of 7 HTA reports on ultra-orphan diseases	All 7 HTAs (100%) cited RWE for effectiveness, safety, dosing trends, or natural history of the disease.

Abbreviations: AOTMiT, Agency for Health Technology Assessment and Tariff Systems; CEA, Cost-effectiveness analysis; HAS, Haute Autorité de Santé; HTA, health technology assessment; ICER, Institute for Clinical and Economic Review; IQWiG, Institute for Quality and Efficacy in Healthcare; NICE, National Institute for Health and Care Excellence; NSCLC, non-small cell lung cancer; PBAC, Pharmaceutical Benefits Advisory Committee; pCODR, Pan-Canadian Oncology Drug Review; RWE, real-world evidence; SLR, systemic literature review; SMC, Scottish Medicines Consortium; ZIN, Zorginstituut Nederland.

6.5.3 Recent Case Studies of Use of RWE in HTAs

Five case studies illustrate more detailed examples of how RWE is used in practice by payers/HTAs and for value-based pricing/contracting or technology appraisal.

6.5.3.1 Real-World Hospitalization Rate for Value-Based Pricing

In a large clinical trial called PARADIGM-HF, Novartis' Entresto® (sacubitril/valsartan) demonstrated superiority to angiotensin-converting enzyme (ACE) inhibitor enalapril, reducing the risk of heart failure, hospitalization, or cardiovascular death by 20%. Due to competition with low-priced generics, Novartis offered US payers to reduce the price of the drug if the real-world hospitalization rate was lower than the targeted threshold[36].

6.5.3.2 Effectiveness and Adherence in a Real-World Setting

Amgen's PCSK9 Inhibitor Repatha® (evolocumab) is indicated for treatment of hyperlipidemia. In 2017, ICER published a report stating that to meet the revised value-based price benchmark, evolocumab would need to be discounted 85–88% from the current wholesale acquisition cost (WAC) of $14,523 annually. This report and other concerns by payers led to significant challenges for the product's pricing and formulary access. Amgen agreed to fully refund the cost of Repatha if in the real-world setting a patient is adherent to the medication and has a heart attack or stroke[37]. Due to payer backlash, the price of the drug was also reduced by 60%[38].

6.5.3.3 Real-World Overall Survival for Managed Access Entry

In Australia, PBAC had granted coverage for ipilimumab for metastatic melanoma with the condition to generate evidence for 2-year overall survival in the real-world setting. Based on the data from 910 patients, the 2-year overall survival was estimated to be between 23.9% and 34.2%, which was higher than the overall survival of 23.5% observed in the key ipilimumab registrational trial[39].

6.5.3.4 Comparator Efficacy in a Real-World Setting

For products that are approved based on non-comparative trials (e.g., single-arm studies for oncology), it can be useful to generate data on efficacy of comparators using real-world studies. For the NICE assessment of brentuximab vedotin for Hodgkin lymphoma, a rare cancer, Takeda Pharmaceuticals leveraged RWE for historical controls, which were used for demonstrating relative effectiveness of the product[40]. The real-world historical control also was used for brentuximab vedotin's assessment in relapsed or refractory systemic anaplastic large cell lymphoma (ALCL). An indirect comparison of brentuximab vedotin to chemotherapy was conducted for progression-free survival and overall survival data for a historical cohort of patients in the British Columbia Cancer Agency Lymphoid Cancer database[41]. A NICE appraisal was done of nivolumab for rrHL. The manufacturer leveraged a previous US retrospective chart review study for demonstrating the efficacy of the comparator. Although NICE had some concerns in using a US study for the United Kingdom, the HTA committee accepted the RWE for the comparator for conducting indirect comparison to nivolumab[27].

6.5.3.5 Natural History of the Disease and Long-Term Effectiveness for Ultra-Orphan Products

For NICE's appraisal of asfotase alfa for pediatric-onset hypophosphatasia, the manufacturer submitted data from three non-interventional real-world natural history studies to demonstrate evidence on survival, need for invasive ventilation, and functional assessments. Additionally, for effectiveness, evidence from two extension studies in a real-world setting was submitted as part of the appraisal.[27]

References

1. Augustovski, F. and McClellan, M.B. 2019. Current policy and practice for value-based pricing. *Value in Health*, 22, S4–S6.
2. Touchot, N. amd Flume, M. 2015. The payers' perspective on gene therapies. *Nature Biotechnology*, 33, 902.
3. Carr, D.R. and Bradshaw, S.E. 2016. Gene therapies: the challenge of super-high-cost treatments and how to pay for them. *Regenerative Medicine*, 11, 381–393.
4. Malone, D.C., et al. 2019. Cost-effectiveness analysis of using onasemnogene abeparvovec (AVXS-101) in spinal muscular atrophy type 1 patients. *Journal of Market Access & Health Policy* 7, 1601484.
5. Danzon, P.M. 2018. Affordability challenges to value-based pricing: mass diseases, orphan diseases, and cures. *Value in Health*, 21, 252–257.
6. Schuller, Y., Hollak, C.E.M., Gispen-de Wied, C.C., Stoyanova-Beninska, V., and Biegstraaten, M. 2017. Factors contributing to the efficacy-effectiveness gap in the case of orphan drugs for metabolic diseases. *Drugs*, 77, 1461–1472.
7. Dafny, L.S., Ody, C.J., and Schmitt, M.A. 2016. Undermining value-based purchasing—lessons from the pharmaceutical industry. *New England Journal of Medicine*, 375, 2013–2015.
8. Mahendraratnam, N., et al. 2019. Value-based arrangements may be more prevalent than assumed. *The American Journal of Managed Care*, 25, 70–76.

9. Jansen, J., Incerti, D., and Linthicum, M. 2017. An open-source consensus-based approach to value assessment. Health Affairs Blog. https://www. healthaffairs. org/do/10.1377/hblog20171212.640960/full/

10. Willke, R.J., Neumann, P.J., Garrison Jr, L.P., and Ramsey, S.D. 2018. Review of recent US value frameworks—a health economics approach: an ISPOR Special Task Force report [6]. *Value in Health*, 21, 155–160.

11. Yu, J.S., Chin, L., Oh, J., and Farias, J. 2017. Performance-based risk-sharing arrangements for pharmaceutical products in the United States: a systematic review. *Journal of Managed Care & Specialty Pharmacy*, 23, 1028–1040.

12. Gonçalves, F.R., Santos, S., Silva, C., and Sousa, G. 2018. Risk-sharing agreements, present and future. *ecancermedicalscience* 12, 823.

13. Duhig, A.M., Saha, S., Smith, S., Kaufman, S., and Hughes, J. 2018. The current status of outcomes-based contracting for manufacturers and payers: an AMCP Membership Survey. *Journal of Managed Care & Specialty Pharmacy*, 24, 410–415.

14. Cieply, B. and Enev, T. 2018. PHP350-performance and outcomes based contracts in the EU and USA: comparison of trends and recent developments. *Value in Health*, 21, S210.

15. Kelly, C. 2016. US outcomes-based contracts: big uptick in interest, but not execution. *In Vivo*, 6, November.

16. Yoo, S.L., et al. 2019. Improving patient access to new drugs in South Korea: evaluation of the National Drug Formulary System. *International Journal of Environmental Research and Public Health*, 16, 288.

17. Department of Health & Human Services. 2019 Transmittal and Notice of Approval of State Plan Material for: Centers for Medicare & Medicaid Services. https://www.medicaid.gov/State-resource-center/Medicaid-State-Plan-Amendments/Downloads/LA/LA-19-0018.pdf

18. Horvath, J.C. and Anderson, G.F. 2019. The states as important laboratories for federal prescription drug cost-containment efforts. *JAMA*, 321, 1561–1562.

19. Hodgson, J., Zec, H., and Bedell, W. 2019. Sell'n gene therapies. *Transfusion*, 1, 20192.

20. Novartis. 2019. AveXis Announces Innovative Zolgensma® Gene Therapy Access Programs for US Payers and Families. https://www.prnewswire.com/news-releases/avexis-announces-innovative-zolgensma-gene-therapy-access-programs-for-us-payers-and-families-300856661.html#:~:text=AveXis%20Announces%20Innovative%20Zolgensma%C2%AE%20Gene%20Therapy%20Access%20Programs,chronic%20therapy%20for%20all%20pediatric%20patients%20with%20SMA

21. Brockelmann, P.J., et al. 2017. Brentuximab vedotin in patients with relapsed or refractory Hodgkin lymphoma who are Ineligible for autologous stem cell transplant: a Germany and United Kingdom retrospective study. *European Journal of Haematology*, 99, 553–558.

22. California Technology Assessment Forum. 2015. Next Steps for Payers and Policymakers: An Action Guide on the Newest Treatments for Chronic Hepatitis C Infection. https://icer-review.org/wp-content/uploads/2016/02/HCV2_action_guide_payers_Final.pdf

23. Optum. 2017. Optum and Merck Collaborate to Advance Value-Based Contracting of Pharmaceuticals. https://www.optum.com/about/news/optum-merck-collaborate-advance-value-based-contracting-pharmaceuticals.html

24. Malone, D.C., Brown, M., Hurwitz, J.T., Peters, L., and Graff, J.S. 2018. Real-world evidence: useful in the real world of US payer decision making? How? When? And what studies? *Value Health*, 21, 326–333.

25. Horberg, M.A., et al. 2018. Association of raltegravir use with long-term health outcomes in HIV-infected patients: an observational post-licensure safety study in a large integrated healthcare system. *HIV Clinical Trials*, 19, 177–187.

26. Joshi, K., et al. 2018. Adherence and economic impact of paliperidone palmitate versus oral atypical antipsychotics in a Medicare population. *Journal of Comparative Effectiveness Research*, 7, 723–735.

27. Aggarwal, S. and Topaloglu, O. 2019. Real-World Evidence: Strategies, Trends, Methods, Case Studies. (CreateSpace Publishing Platform ISBN 9781719037068).

28. Ng, C., et al. 2018. Resource utilization and cost of influenza requiring hospitalization in Canadian adults: A study from the serious outcomes surveillance network of the Canadian Immunization Research Network. *Influenza and Other Respiratory Viruses*, 12, 232–240.

29. ICER Institute for Clinical and Economic Review. 2018. Inotersen and Patisiran for Hereditary Transthyretin Amylooidosis: Effectiveness and Value. Final Evidence Report. https://icer-review.org/wp-content/uploads/2018/02/ICER_Amyloidosis_Final_Evidence_Report_100418.pdf

30. Makady, A., et al. 2018. Using real-world data in Health Technology Assessment (HTA) practice: a comparative study of five HTA agencies. *Pharmacoeconomics*, 36, 359–368.

31. Drane, E., Upton, E., Morten, P., and Walker, E. 2019. PNS182-Real-world evidence on the rise: evaluating the use of real-world evidence in ICER assessments of comparative clinical effectiveness. *Value in Health*, 22, S316.

32. Ng, T., Chawla, T., and Bending, M. 2018. PCN293-What is the value of real world evidence in oncology in HTA appraisals in England, France, Canada and Australia? *Value in Health*, 21, S64.

33. Aggarwal, S., Topaloglu, O., and Kumar, S. 2018. Using real-world evidence for health technology assessment submissions: lessons and insights from Review of Nice's Technology Assessment Reports (2016-2017). *Value in Health*, 21, S7.

34. Han, D., Tiruneh, M., Chambers, A., and Haynes, A. 2018. VP02 real-world evidence (RWE) and CADTH Pan-Canadian Oncology Drug Review. *International Journal of Technology Assessment in Health Care*, 34, 159–160.

35. Wilk, N., et al. 2017. Study types and reliability of real world evidence compared with experimental evidence used in Polish reimbursement decision-making processes. *Public Health*, 145, 51–58.

36. Walker, T. 2016. Novartis signs on to value-based pricing for Entresto. *Managed HealthCare Executive*, 4, May.

37. Kee, A. and Maio, V. 2019. Value-based contracting: challenges and opportunities. *American Journal of Medical Quality*, 34, 615–617.

38. Robinson, J.G., et al. 2019. Enhancing the value of PCSK9 monoclonal antibodies by identifying patients most likely to benefit. *Journal of Clinical Lipidology*, 13, 525–537.

39. Kim, H., Comey, S., Hausler, K., and Cook, G. 2018. A real world example of coverage with evidence development in Australia - ipilimumab for the treatment of metastatic melanoma. *Journal of Pharmaceutical Policy and Practice*, 11, 4.

40. National Institute for Ehalth and Care Excellence. 2018. Brentuximab vedotin for treating CD30-positive Hodgkin lymphoma. Technology Appraisal Guidance. https://www.nice.org.uk/guidance/ta524/resources/brentuximab-vedotin-for-treating-cd30positive-hodgkin-lymphoma-pdf-82606840474309
41. National Institute for Ehalth and Care Excellence. 2017. Brentuximab vedotin for Treating Relapsed or Refractory Systemic Anaplastic Large Cell Lymphoma. https://www.nice.org.uk/guidance/ta478/chapter/3-Committee-discussion.

7

Causal Inference for Observational Studies/Real-World Data

Bo Lu

7.1 Causal Inference with Real-World Data

Inferring causal effects has been the perennial effort in many scientific fields, including health, medicine, epidemiology, economics, statistics, computer science, sociology, political science, and so forth. The rigorous pursuit of causal inference was made possible after Neyman (1990) proposed the basic idea of the potential outcome framework. Rubin (1974) further formalized the framework that sets the stage for statistical inference on causal effects. For a binary treatment (i.e., taking the drug vs. not taking the drug), each individual can present two potential outcomes, one under each possible treatment scenario. Denoting the pair of potential outcomes as (Y^1, Y^0), where 1 indicates taking the drug and 0 for not taking the drug, we can define causal effects at different levels clearly, for example:

- Individual causal effect: $Y_i^1 - Y_i^0$, for individual i.
- Population average treatment effect (PATE): $E(Y^1 - Y^0)$, for the entire study population.
- Subpopulation average treatment effect: $E(Y^1 - Y^0 \mid X)$, for a specific subpopulation defined by covariate X.

As the name suggests, potential outcomes are not something that we can always observe in reality. We can only see one outcome as the participant goes through one specific treatment arm. It turns out to be a missing data problem as at least one of the two potential outcomes is not recorded in causal inference. Therefore, the causal effect identification needs more assumptions than what are usually required for estimating the associational effects in common statistical analysis. Typically, the following two assumptions are used:

- Stable unit treatment value assumption (SUTVA): It has two implications. First, the treatment applied to one unit does not affect the outcome for other units. This no interference requirement may hold true for a conventional drug study, where we do not expect individual drug-taking behavior to have any impact on other people's outcomes. But it may not be valid in other scenarios, such as vaccination studies, where the efficacy of the vaccine depends on how many people in the population actually receive it. Second, an individual receiving a specific treatment level cannot receive different forms of that treatment. This assumption guarantees that there is only one version for each treatment being compared. In a controlled trial, this is likely to hold. But in some longitudinal studies with potential noncompliance, individuals assigned to the same treatment group may be exposed to the drug at various cumulative doses, then it might be questionable to assume that they always receive the identical treatment.

- Ignorable treatment assignment: It assumes that the probability of receiving treatment should be strictly between 0 and 1 for each individual, and whether a unit gets the treatment or not does not depend on his or her potential outcomes, provided that all relevant covariates are controlled for.

It is evident that the ignorability assumption holds under a randomized allocation, because the treatment assignment does not depend on any covariate. If we can add more design features, such as "doubly blinded" and "controlled," to a randomized study, the SUTVA is more likely to hold. Then we can confidently estimate the treatment effect via a randomized controlled trial. Observational study is an empirical investigation to elucidate cause-and-effect relationships, when random allocation of treatment is not feasible (Rosenbaum 2017). Clearly, the ignorability of treatment assignment breaks down, which makes the confounding control a challenging task. It consists of two parts: (1) control of measured confounding (overt bias), as important observed covariates may be distributed differently between two arms prior to the treatment, and (2) control of unmeasured confounding (hidden bias), as not all relevant covariates are observed in observational studies. Statistical methodology for the former has been well established and recognized; however, the methods for the latter have been much less utilized, though available.

Randomized experiment is seemingly a perfect tool for causal inference, but its utility is rather limited for the following reasons: First, because it is conducted in a restrictive manner with selected participants, it is hard to generalize the findings to the target population. Second, it may be time consuming and resource craving, especially for large randomized clinical trials. Third, there is no guarantee that the study will be executed perfectly. Any violation to the protocol, such as loss of follow-up or noncompliance, may make the randomized study more or less like an observational one. Last, it is not possible to run randomized studies to answer all causal question, i.e., evaluation of healthcare system or health policy, the impact of off-label drug use, and so forth. The lack of depth and breadth of causal inference with randomized studies in many situations brings the use of observational data to the front stage.

Causal inference with non-experimental data has a long history. One of the most famous examples is the debate on whether smoking causes lung cancer in 1950s and 1960s. Apparently, the randomized controlled trial is not a suitable design due to ethical and practical reasons. Researchers had to rely on evidence generated from observational data to elucidate the relationship. Despite a myriad of studies showing strong association between smoking and lung cancer, supporters of a non-causal relationship argued that (1) association does not imply causation, (2) there may be a genetic predisposition to both smoking and lung cancer, and (3) a few studies showed a beneficial association of smoking (low lung cancer incidence in the smoker group). In 1959, Cornfield et al. (1959) joined with five leading cancer experts and wrote a paper that surveyed many published studies, examined the objections from some famous statisticians and tobacco companies, provided a carefully reasoned account of the controversy, and showed how the evidence was overwhelmingly in favor of showing that "smoking is a causative factor in the rapidly increasing incidence of human epidermoid carcinoma of the lung." The 1964 General Surgeon's Report on smoking and health "highlighted the deleterious health consequences of tobacco use" and put an end to the decades-long debate (Centers for Disease Control and Prevention [CDC] 2006). Starting the following year, Congress required all cigarette packages distributed in the United States to carry a health warning message.

Even in the fields that used to be dominated by randomized controlled trials, such as drug and medical device development, the landscape begins to change in the modern era of big data. In 2016, Congress passed the 21st Century Cures Act (2006), which included provisions requiring the U.S. Food and Drug Administration (FDA) to evaluate the potential use of real-world evidence (RWE). RWE is generally defined as "data regarding the usage, or the potential benefits or risks, of a drug derived from sources other than randomized clinical trials." It opens the door for research effort using a wide range of data, including medical records, health records, registry data, claims data, surveys, administrative database, and so forth.

In 2017, the FDA moved forward with approving a new indication for a medical device without requiring any new clinical trials. A transcatheter aortic valve replacement (TAVR) is a minimally invasive surgical procedure that repairs the damaged valve without removing it. FDA approved the use of the first TAVR device, the Edwards Sapien transcatheter heart valve (THV), for patients with severe symptoms but are too risky for surgery in 2011. Since then, the device manufacturer had established a product registry with over 100,000 TAVR records. Among these records were 600 records relating to the then off-label use of the new procedure, the Sapien 3. Based on the product registry data, FDA approved use of the new procedure without requiring costly and time-consuming randomized clinical trials. This approval represents a significant milestone in expanded use of RWE in regulatory drug and medical device development (Belson 2018).

The chapter is organized as follows: Section 7.2 reviews various strategies of propensity score adjustment in observational studies, Section 7.3 introduces the sensitivity analysis to assess the impact due a potentially unmeasured confounder, and Section 4 presents an example using real-world data to evaluate the U.S. trauma care system.

7.2 Propensity Score Adjustment for Observational Studies

Observational studies attempt to estimate the treatment effects by comparing outcomes for subjects who are not randomly assigned to treatment and control groups. In the modern era of big data, the sources for observational data are abundant, including administrative records, registries, electronic health records, claim databases, surveys, and so forth. Without a random assignment mechanism, some subjects are more likely than others to receive the treatment due to differences in individual characteristics (e.g., age, gender, disease severity), in observational studies. Therefore, careful statistical adjustments are needed to justify the causal interpretation based on the analysis of observational data. It is clear that the assignment mechanism is broken in observational studies due to the lack of randomization, so it is natural to devise tools to fix this broken link. The propensity score, defined as the conditional probability of exposure to a treatment given observed covariates, is a technical tool that addresses the treatment assignment problem. It can balance the observed covariate distributions between treatment and non-treatment groups and thus approximate a randomization-like scenario in terms of treatment assignment. Thus, propensity score methods can reduce the covariates-induced bias in treatment effect estimation (Rosenbaum and Rubin 1983a).

Formally, denoting T as a dichotomous treatment indicator (1 for being treated and 0 for being untreated) and X as the vector of observed covariates, we may define the propensity score $e(X)$ as:

$$e(X) = Pr(T = 1 | X)$$

Propensity scores are typically used in a nonparametric form to remove the observed confounding bias, such as, constructing matched pairs, serving as selection weights, or creating homogeneous strata. If the structural relationship between the outcome and some covariates is known, propensity scores can be combined with regression adjustment to improve the estimation efficiency. The rest of this subsection provides more details about different ways of using propensity scores analytically.

7.2.1 Propensity Score Matching

Matching refers to classifying subjects into small groups so that there are both treated and untreated subjects in each group and they are similar in terms of matching variables. Matching on propensity scores closely resembles a block randomized design, where the treatment assignment is random within each subgroup. Generally, propensity score matching is considered advantageous in the following perspectives. (1) It is more robust in the sense that it uses a nonparametric way to balance the covariate distributions between treated and untreated groups, which does not rely on parametric outcome models. (2) It resembles the randomization design, which is easily interpretable to a general audience. (3) It is more objective in the sense that the causal effect inference is conducted only after good matches are established and the outcome variable never enters the matching process. (4) Matching-based sensitivity analysis is well developed to assess the impact of hidden bias.

Ideally, we want to match exactly on every single covariate to remove the observed confounding. But this is often impossible in practice, especially when there are a large number of covariates. The propensity score is considered as a dimension reduction tool because it is a scalar and matching it can remove all biases related to treatment assignment under the ignorability assumption (Rosenbaum and Rubin 1983a). To successfully implement matching to infer causal relationship, we need to carefully consider the design and algorithm, assess the covariate balance after matching, select inferential procedures compatible with matching structure, and conduct the sensitivity analysis. We will go over each of them briefly in this subsection (except the sensitivity analysis, which will be covered in the next section). For a more detailed description of matching, readers may refer to Stuart (2010).

7.2.1.1 Matching Design

Matching group subjects into well-structured matched sets and such structure may play a role in determining the statistical inference procedure. Each set must contain subjects from both treated and control groups for comparison purposes. Matching design refers to the structure generated from the matching process. There are three general types of design: bipartite matching, non-bipartite matching. and poly-matching (Figure 7.1).

Bipartite matching is the most commonly seen design. It is used when there are two well-defined treatment groups (i.e., treated vs. control), and matching is always conducted between the two groups. If one treated subject is matched to one control subject, this is known as a pair match. If one treated subject is matched to a fixed number of k ($k > 1$) control subjects, often used to improve the efficiency of the estimation, it is known as a 1-k match. A variation to 1-k match is called a variable match, where one treated subject can be matched to multiple controls, but the ratio is not pre-fixed to achieve better matching quality. To further improve the matching quality, a full matching

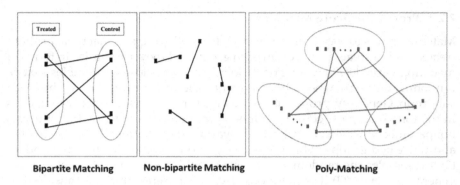

Bipartite Matching   **Non-bipartite Matching**   **Poly-Matching**

FIGURE 7.1
Three types of matching designs

design may be considered, which allows one treated subject matched to multiple controls or the other way around (Rosenbaum 1991).

When there are multiple exposure groups or there is no clearly defined two groups, non-bipartite matching is used to form pair structure between any two groups when appropriate. It can create matched pairs with multiple dose-level groups that maximize dose difference within the pair to explore potential treatment effects. It also may be used in longitudinal data matching to find best matches across different timepoints. Interested readers may refer to Lu et al (2011) for further details.

Poly-matching is a new design focusing on creating matched sets with one subject from each group, when there are more than two exposure groups. It provides a simple and clean structure to make statistical inference among multiple treatment groups, as it represents a block randomization design well. An example of matching with three exposure groups, namely triplet matching, can be found in (Nattino et al. 2019).

7.2.1.2 Matching Algorithm

As a computational procedure, matching requires a special algorithm. The simplest way is via a nearest neighbor algorithm. It randomly sorts the groups, then creates pairs by finding the ones with the closest distance. It is easy to implement, but the greedy nature may produce matched sets with a very large total distance, which may compromise the overall matching quality. To improve the matching distance globally, we can consider the optimal matching algorithm, which minimizes the total distance of matched pairs among all possible parings. The optimal algorithms are available for both bipartite and non-bipartite matching in selected software packages. The optimal solution for poly-matching is not available as it goes beyond a pair-match structure. Nattino et al. (2020) proposed a conditional three-way algorithm for triplet matching, which is shown to obtain a total distance no more than twofold the optimal result. The idea can be extended to more than three groups.

7.2.1.3 Post-Matching Balance Checking

An important difference of matching from the traditional regression adjustment of covariates is that we need to check the covariate balance after matching. Regression adjustment relies on the parametric functional form to adjust for covariate imbalance, which may introduce bias if the functional form is mis-specified. Matching achieves the balance nonparametrically by pairing similar subjects together. Well-matched subjects reduce the bias introduced by observed covariates. Rubin (2001) provided three distributional conditions that a good regression adjustment should satisfy, which can be used as a guideline for post-matching balance checking. From a practical perspective, we usually check the covariate mean differences via standardized differences and the variance difference via logarithm of standard deviation ratio for each covariate, both before and after matching.

7.2.1.4 Post-Matching Inference

There are two different views on how to perform post-matching inference. Though both regard matching as a means to re-create a randomization-like scenario, they differ in how to use the randomization distribution and whether the matching structure should be accounted for in the analysis.

The traditional statistical view tries to take advantage of the randomization distribution of the treatment assignment. Well-matched pairs are considered as coming from a block randomization design. Within each pair, both subjects have the same probability of receiving the treatment and only one of them gets it. Suppose there are n matched pairs, denote Ω be the set containing all possible values of treatment assignment, then for any possible assignment t,

$$\Pr\left(T = t \mid \text{matching}\right) = \frac{1}{|\Omega|} = \frac{1}{2^n}, \text{ for all } \in \Omega.$$

This constitutes a randomization distribution under the ignorability assumption. For any test statistics $S = s(T, Y)$, we can test the causal null hypothesis without additional distribution assumption. A commonly seen null hypothesis of causal effect is the Fisher's sharp null hypothesis, $H_0 : Y^1 = Y^0$. Interested readers may refer to Rosenbaum (2002) for more discussion on causal null hypotheses. The major advantage of this randomization-based inference is the robustness to potentially mis-specify outcome models. But this may come at the price of statistical efficiency, or not making full use of covariate information. If an outcome model is well justified, we may consider regression analysis accounting for paired structure, i.e., conditional logistic regression (CLR) for binary outcome, stratified Cox proportional hazards model for survival data, and so forth (Austin 2014)

A more empirical view ignores the matching structure in the analysis (Ho et al. 2007). It regards matching as a nonparametric data pre-processing step, which creates a situation similar to a complete randomization design. It is sensible in complex observational studies with a large number of covariates. When the dimension is high, matching may only balance the covariates at a group level, rather than within each pair. Matching on propensity score only warrants removing bias along the propensity score direction, not necessarily for every single covariate. Therefore, post-matching analysis accounting for the matching structure may not be as advantageous. The main critic is that this strategy is somewhat ad hoc, with a lack of theoretical justification.

7.2.2 Propensity Score Weighting

Weighting is another popular way for propensity score adjustment. The original idea comes from survey sampling literature, i.e., the Hortivz-Thompson estimator, as we can view the inverse of propensity score as a sampling weight of selecting subjects to treatment. It has been shown that the PATE can be estimated unbiasedly using propensity score weighting:

$$\text{PATE} = E\left(Y^1\right) - E\left(Y^0\right) = E\left[\frac{Y1_{T=1}}{e(X)}\right] - E\left[\frac{Y1_{T=0}}{1-e(X)}\right]$$

For treated subjects, the weight is the inverse of the propensity score and for control subjects, the weight is the inverse of one-minus-the-propensity-score. The use of weights is to create a pseudo-population in which all covariates are balanced at the population level. Then confounding is no longer an issue in causal effect estimation.

From a practical perspective, the propensity score is not known in advance and researchers must estimate it. Whether using parametric or nonparametric methods, there is always a chance that the propensity score is not estimated correctly. This is less an issue for matching because the estimated propensity score itself does not go into the estimator. As long as the matching obtains desirable balance, it should be fine for the design purpose, but the situation is different for weighting, as the estimated propensity score is part of the estimator. A mis-specified propensity score model will introduce substantial bias. To overcome this, researchers have developed a so-called "doubly robust" estimation strategy, which combines the propensity score and a regression model to improve the performance (Bang and Robins 2005). A regression model on the outcome is introduced to guard against potential mis-specifications of the propensity score model. Such a model is known as a structural model to differentiate from the conventional regression model, because it models the potential outcomes rather than the observed ones. A common type of structural model is the marginal structural model, which focuses on the marginal causal effect (Robins et al. 2000). The advantage of the doubly robust estimation strategy is that it has two chances to get a consistent estimate of the causal effect: (1) when the outcome model is incorrectly specified but the propensity score model is correctly specified or (2) when the propensity score model is incorrectly specified but the outcome model is correctly specified. When both models are correct, it yields an efficient causal effect estimator (Tan 2007).

7.2.3 Propensity Score Stratification

Stratification refers to the procedure that groups subjects by similar propensity score values, which follows the idea of block randomization. If the propensity score values are pretty homogeneous within each stratum, we can effectively remove confounding bias by first doing stratum-level causal effect estimation, then combining across all strata. It is easier to implement than matching or weighting, as it does not require special algorithms or statistical computational procedures to handle weights. Depending on the sample size, researchers may divide the data into 5 or 10 groups (or even more if the sample size allows). One key step is to make sure that there are enough treated and control subjects within each stratum to warrant a valid estimation of stratum-specific causal effect.

One major issue is that propensity score stratification is often not good enough to remove confounding by itself. Just grouping subjects into a few strata may lead to residual confounding within each stratum. So additional covariate adjustment is highly recommended (Imbens and Rubin 2015).

Overall, all three strategies have seen ample applications. Matching follows the randomization design principle more closely, which is especially good for non-model-based inference. Weighting can be combined with models more naturally, which also enjoys the doubly robust property. Stratification can be viewed as a coarsened matching design or a special weighting strategy. Its main advantage is simplicity, which may be used by those with limited statistical background.

7.3 Sensitivity Analysis for Hidden Bias

The key assumption of the propensity score adjustment is the treatment assignment ignorability. However, in observational studies, there is usually the concern that some important baseline covariates were not measured, so merely adjusting for observed covariates is not enough to remove all confounding biases. Therefore, sensitivity analysis is introduced to address the question: What would the unmeasured covariate have to be like to alter the conclusions of the study (Rosenbaum 2005)?

The first sensitivity analysis was conducted by Cornfield et al. (1959) to study the potential impact of cigarette smoking on lung cancer incidence. As part of the argument by the tobacco industry and others who had questioned smoking as a causal agent of lung cancer, they claimed that some other unobserved difference between smokers and non-smokers, i.e., something genetic in origin, may be the cause. Cornfield et al. (1959) found that, to rule out cigarette smoking as a cause of lung cancer completely, such an unobserved characteristic would need to be about nine times more common among smokers than among nonsmokers. It also would need to have a nearly perfect correlation with lung cancer status, which was considered impossible by clinical experts.

There are various methods for sensitivity analysis in observational data (Lin et al. 1998; Robins et al. 1999; Imbens 2003; Ding and VanderWeele 2016). In this chapter, we focus on approaches following Cornfield's idea, which was later formalized by Rosenbaum and Rubin (1983b). This sensitivity analysis was developed based on matched design with a randomization inference framework, which does not need additional modeling assumptions. But it could be quite computationally intensive for large data sets often encountered in RWE research. Recently, Nattino and Lu (2018) extended such a sensitivity analysis by introducing a simple outcome model. It simplifies the calculation substantially and provides a closed-form solution to the sensitivity parameter boundary corresponding to non-significant causal effects. More importantly, in a large sample, it yields the same results as the conventional sensitivity analysis.

7.3.1 The Setup of Sensitivity Analysis

To account for the hidden bias, a binary indicator U is introduced as a proxy for the unmeasured confounder. With U, we restore the ignorability of treatment assignment:

$$\left(Y^1, Y^0\right) \perp T \mid X, U$$

To incorporate the impact of U on treatment assignment, a logistic regression model is considered:

$$logit\left[Pr\left(T_i = 1 \mid X_i, U_i\right)\right] = \kappa(X_i) + \gamma U_i$$

Without loss of generality, X and U are assumed to be independent; $\kappa(X_i)$ is a nuisance part representing the impact due to observed covariates and it would be balanced by matching; and $\Gamma = e^\gamma \geq 1$ is known as the sensitivity parameter. When $\Gamma = 1$, this is the conventional propensity score model and there is no unmeasured confounding. When $\Gamma > 1$, hidden bias is present. Even within well-matched pairs on X, the treatment assignment probabilities may still differ if their U values are different. Technically, Γ captures the association between treatment reception and U in the odds ratio scale. For example, if $\Gamma = 2$, two units in the matched pair that appear similar with regards to the observed covariates, X, could differ in their odds of receiving the treatment by as much as a factor of 2. Then, one of them might be twice (in the odds ratio scale) as likely as the other to receive the treatment, due to the unmeasured factor. If this factor also is related to the outcome, the "calculated" treatment effect with adjustment only for observed covariates might be mitigated if U is accounted for.

The sensitivity analysis tries to answer the question: How large must Γ be to alter the conclusion based on the observed data qualitatively? That is, the qualitative conclusion of the study will change from significant to insignificant. A study is highly sensitive to hidden bias if the conclusion changes for Γ are just barely greater than 1, and it is robust or insensitive if the conclusion changes only for quite large values of Γ (Rosenbaum 2005).

7.3.2 Sensitivity Analysis Based on Randomization Inference

Rosenbaum (2002) provided a detailed description of the theoretical development for sensitivity analysis based on matched designs. Suppose we first match treated and control subjects using the propensity score. With well-matched pairs, we may conduct a Wilcoxon signed rank test for continuous outcomes, McNemar's test for binary outcomes, or paired Prentice-Wilcoxon (PPW) test for survival outcomes (Lu et al. 2018). All these tests belong to a general class of test statistics, known as the sign score statistics. Under the Fisher's sharp null hypothesis, both potential outcomes are known and the only random thing is the treatment assignment. Therefore, the sign score statistic can be written as the sum of a series of independent Bernoulli random variables. When hidden bias is present, the probability distribution for each Bernoulli variable depends on U, which is not known. But it is unknown only to a finite degree measured by Γ. For the test statistic of the causal effect, Rosenbaum (2002) derived the bounding distributions that are functions of Γ. Then, for each fixed $\Gamma \geq 1$, the sensitivity analysis computes the bounds for p-values of the test. For $\Gamma = 1$, there is only a single p-value as a randomized study since U does not enter the equation. For $\Gamma > 1$, one can calculate an upper bound and a lower bound of the p-values, or a range of p-values, to account for the potential impact of U. As Γ increases, reflecting more uncertainty about the impact of U, the range becomes wider, and eventually, it becomes too wide and passes a certain threshold for inferential purpose, i.e., p-value greater than 0.05. The tipping point, Γ, at which it passes the threshold is reported as a measure for sensitivity to hidden bias.

There are other variations of such sensitivity analysis. The original one focusing on the impact of U on the treatment assignment is referred to as primal sensitivity analysis. The dual sensitivity analysis focuses on the impact of U on the outcome. A third one that incorporates U's impact on both the treatment assignment and the outcome is known as simultaneous sensitivity analysis. Because the confounder is a variable that affects both treatment and outcome, the simultaneous sensitivity analysis provides a complete picture of how the hidden bias with varying magnitudes may change the conclusion qualitatively. For a binary outcome, a logistic regression model is used to incorporate the potential impact due to U:

$$logit\left[Pr\left(Y_i = 1 \mid X_i, U_i\right)\right] = \xi\left(X_i\right) + \delta U_i$$

where $\Delta = e^{\delta}$ is a second sensitivity parameter representing the impact of U on the outcome.

In fact, the primal sensitivity analysis is a more conservative special case of the simultaneous sensitivity analysis, as it reflects the situation when the impact of U on the outcome is extremely large (Gastwirth et al. 1998).

When the sample size is small, p-values for randomization inference are not too hard to compute. With large sample sizes, Rosenbaum recommended using normal approximation to the test statistics to facilitate the calculation. The implementation of the conventional sensitivity analysis can be tedious, especially for the simultaneous sensitivity analysis, because there is no closed-form solution to the tipping point values of Γ and Δ.

7.3.3 Model-Assisted Sensitivity Analysis

The model-assisted sensitivity analysis aims to simplify the computation and to provide a conceptually easier interpretation. This sensitivity analysis also is based on a matched design. After matching, instead of doing a randomization test, one can use a CLR model to test the causal effect for a binary outcome:

$$logit\left[Pr\left(Y_{si} = 1 \mid T_{si}\right)\right] = \alpha_s + \beta T_{si}$$

where matched sets are represented by s, and we assume a constant treatment effect across all matched sets, β.

The causal effect null hypothesis based on this model is $H_0 : \beta = 0$. It is slightly weaker than the Fisher's sharp null hypothesis used in the conventional sensitivity analysis. It requires homogeneous unity odds ratios for treated versus untreated groups under the null, rather than identical potential outcomes.

A key insight for the model-assisted sensitivity analysis is that to reach the upper bound of the p-value for the causal effect test, the unmeasured confounder U needs to be perfectly associated with Y (i.e., $U = Y$). In other words, under the null hypothesis of the no treatment effect, if we fix the association between the lurking factor and the treatment, its largest effect on the causal effect test is attained in the worst-case scenario where the unobserved factor perfectly predicts the outcome. If the treatment has no effect, the lurking factor can at most produce a spurious causal effect with a magnitude of Γ. If we observe any association more than Γ, at least part of it must come from the true treatment effect.

Nattino and Lu (2018) showed that the score test in CLR is asymptotically equivalent to the McNemar's test used in the conventional sensitivity analysis. Therefore, the two sensitivity analyses yield the same results in large samples. Denoting the conditional odds ratio of treatment effect as $OR_C(Z,Y)$, they also established the link between the upper bound of the *p*-values computed in the conventional sensitivity analysis and the *p*-value of the one-sided test about the conditional effect, that is, $H_0 : OR_C(Z,Y) = \Gamma$ versus the alternative $H_a : OR_C(Z,Y) > \Gamma$. Denote with Ω^+ the set of sensitivity parameter values that correspond to the *p*-value upper bounds exceeding the significance level of the test, α. Then the set can be described as the collection of parameters Γ such that the *p*-value of the above test is non-significant, which is just the one-sided $(1-\alpha)100\%$ confidence interval of $OR_C(Z,Y)$.

The model-assisted sensitivity analysis provides a more accurate account of the magnitude of the unmeasured confounder needed to explain away the observed finding. Cornfield et al. (1959) claimed that the unobserved characteristic would need to be about nine times more common among smokers than among nonsmokers, given an observed ninefold risk difference. If this were in odds ratio scale, the unmeasured characteristic needs to be at the lower bound of the one-sided confidence interval of $OR_C(Z,Y)$, which should be smaller than nine, to wipe out the observed effect.

The CLR model used in the sensitivity analysis is just for testing purposes in a matched setup. It does not posit any structure relationship between the outcome and covariates, because no covariate enters the model; thus, it is referred as model-assisted rather than model-based. One technical restriction is that it requires homogenous conditional odds ratios, and more work is needed to extend the idea to continuous outcomes (Nattino and Lu 2018). The next section will illustrate the detailed implementation of both sensitivity analyses using a real-world dataset on trauma care evaluation.

7.4 Case Study: Propensity Score Matching Design and Sensitivity Analysis for Trauma Care Evaluation

More young Americans die from traumatic injuries—such as car crashes, falls, or homicides—than from any other cause, which makes injury the leading cause of death among persons aged 1 to 44 years old. Trauma centers provide specialized medical services and resources to patients suffering from traumatic injuries. Hospitals in the United States can be categorized as Trauma Center (TC) and Non-Trauma Center (NTC), according to resources and expertise. Patients are admitted to TCs or NTCs depending on various factors, including severity of the injury, geographical restrictions, or other patient characteristics. This is by no means a random process, so the evaluation becomes an RWE study.

Using the 2006–2010 National Emergency Data Sample (NEDS) (Agency for Healthcare Research and Quality 2016), we evaluate the performance of the two levels of trauma care with respect to a key outcome, emergency department (ED) mortality. We consider trauma patients, aged 18–64, characterized by a severe trauma (injury severity score [ISS] ≥25). Detailed description of the data can be found elsewhere (Shi et al. 2016).

The exposure under investigation was the admission to NTCs (vs. TCs) and the binary outcome was ED mortality. The research question was "would the outcome of patients treated at a NTC be different if these patients had been treated at a TC?" The answer to this question has important implications to regional trauma care planning. TCs are supposed to offer the best care to trauma patients, with active research agenda and assuming a leader role in education, but they are also resource craving, which makes them less available in rural areas. A matching design is appropriate to evaluate this causal effect, which corresponds to the exposure effect on the exposed. Our original sample consisted of 21,855 patients, of whom 5314 (24.3%) and 16,541 (75.7%) patients were admitted to NTCs and TCs, respectively. For illustration purposes, we used NTC patients admitted in 2008 (1085) to ensure a large enough pool of available controls for matching design.

7.4.1 Propensity Score Matching

Following Shi et al. (2016), we used the same set of covariates in our propensity score model, which includes age, ISS, chronic conditions, median household income, insurance payer, patient location, multiple injury, and sex. A logistic regression with the NTC indicator as outcome was fitted. Each NTC patient was matched to a TC patient based on the estimated propensity score without replacement, using the optimal matching algorithm (Hansen and Klopfer 2006). As a result, there were 1085 matched pairs with one NTC patient and one TC patient in each pair.

7.4.2 Balance Checking

The major goal of the propensity score adjustment is to recreate a randomization-like scenario where all covariates are balanced between treated and control groups. Such balance effectively removes confounding as covariates are not correlated with the treatment indicator. Therefore, a critical step in matching procedure is to checking covariate balance after matching.

To check the overall balance, we plotted the distributions of the propensity scores in matched NTC and TC groups, which look identical in Figure 7.2. For individual covariate balance, two quantities are usually used for assessing

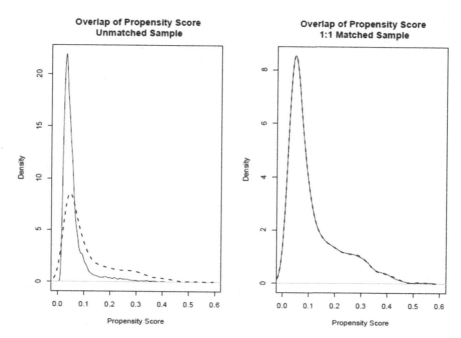

FIGURE 7.2
Overlap of the propensity score before and after matching

balance. The first one is the absolute standardized difference (ASD) for mean balance (Imbens and Rubin 2015). For each continuous covariate, we calculated the absolute mean difference between NTC and TC groups, standardized by the pre-matching pooled standard deviation of the mean (binary outcomes follow a similar formula). The second quantity is the logarithm of the standard deviation ratio between NTC and TC groups for variance balance (Imbens and Rubin 2015). Table 7.1 reports these two measures for each covariate, before and after matching to show the improvement of balance due to matching. As a rule of thumb, we consider 10% or smaller ASDs as a sign of good balance.

In practice, Love's plot is a popular graphical tool for presenting the balance result. Figure 7.3 depicts the absolute standardized mean difference for each variable before and after matching. For all covariates, the ASDs are below 10%, which is considered well balanced. In particular, chronic conditions and multiple injury indicators present large discrepancies before matching and the balance is substantially improved after matching.

7.4.3 Inference Under Ignorability

Because matching achieves good balance for all covariates, as shown in Table 7.1, we can proceed with the outcome analysis to detect the causal

TABLE 7.1

Covariate Balance Before and After Matching

Variable	Standardized Differences		Log Ratio of SD	
	Unmatched	1:1 Match	Unmatched	1:1 Match
Age	8.13	2.93	−0.0121	−0.0105
ISS	4.07	8.40	−0.3345	−0.2298
Chronic conditions	37.72	5.23	−0.0981	−0.0046
Median Household Income by Patient Zip Code				
Q1 (0–25%)	12.68	0.00	0.0530	0.0000
Q2 (25–50%)	4.25	3.27	−0.0203	0.0139
Q3 (50–75%)	4.90	0.67	−0.0336	−0.0043
Q4 (75–100%)	3.17	0.00	-0.0315	0.0000
Primary Expected Payer				
Medicare	5.14	5.94	−0.1069	−0.1261
Medicaid	12.60	3.19	0.1312	−0.0426
Private insurance	7.56	5.54	0.0043	−0.0069
Self-pay	12.06	7.27	−0.0868	0.0399
No charge	3.44	6.56	−0.1323	0.1815
Other	5.98	3.34	−0.0785	0.0378
Patient Location				
Large central metropolitan area	14.85	1.87	0.1150	−0.0183
Large fringe metropolitan area	11.19	3.89	0.0825	−0.0356
Medium metropolitan area	1.55	5.94	−0.0101	0.0348
Small metropolitan area	12.42	4.32	−0.1681	0.0445
Micropolitan area	8.21	0.00	−0.0817	0.0000
Neither metropolitan nor micropolitan area	9.40	4.44	−0.1187	−0.0515
Multiple injury	62.72	0.48	−0.5271	−0.0015
Sex (female)	1.02	2.55	0.0059	0.0144

effect, under the assumption of no unmeasured confounding. With a binary outcome and a paired design, McNemar's test is a natural choice for testing the difference between NTC and TC groups. Table 7.2 summarizes the outcome by TC status and a p-value less than 0.001 is achieved by applying the McNemar's test. This is an easy and clean way to conduct the causal effect testing, as it only relies on matching design to balance all covariates with no modeling involved. As pointed out in Rosenbaum (2010), McNemar's test belongs to a general class of sign score statistics, which is a class of nonparametric statistics based on the randomization distribution of the treatment assignment. Because the sample size is very

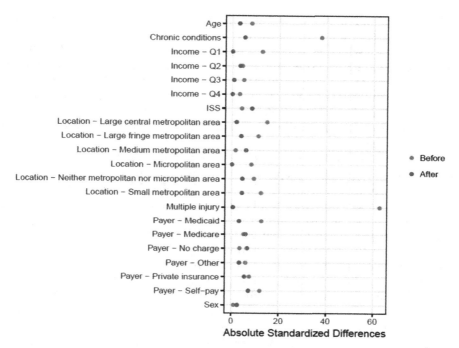

FIGURE 7.3
Love's plot for Absolute Standardized Differences

large here, we use the large sample version of the McNemar's test with a test statistic value of 4.36. In the absence of unmeasured confounding, there is very strong evidence of a mortality difference between being treated at an NTC versus a TC.

7.4.4 Simultaneous Sensitivity Analysis

In the presence of unmeasured confounding, which is likely to be the case for large observational studies, the causal effect test conducted in the previous section might not be valid. We need to account for the impact due to the potential unmeasured confounder to see if the causal effect test is still significant.

TABLE 7.2

Distribution of ED Deaths in Matched Pairs

Trauma Centers	Non-Trauma Centers	
	Death	Alive
Death	25	70
Alive	132	858

To get a complete picture of the impact of unmeasured confounding, we adopted the simultaneous sensitivity analysis. It assumes an unobserved confounder, U, which is associated with the admission to NTC with a magnitude up to $\Gamma \geq 1$ (in odds ratio scale) and is associated with death with a magnitude up to $\Delta \geq 1$ (in odds ratio scale). Then $\Gamma = 1$ and $\Delta = 1$ represents the case when there is no hidden bias. When both $\Gamma > 1$ and $\Delta > 1$, this unobserved confounder would explain away some of the association between NTC admission and mortality, if not all. Then the p-value for the adjusted test should be larger.

Using the conventional simultaneous sensitivity analysis described in Gastwirth et al. (1998), we reported the adjusted p-values of the McNemar's test for different combinations of Γ and Δ in Table 7.3. The varying values of Γ and Δ reflect our uncertainty about the impact due to U. In general, the greater the sensitivity parameters get, the more impact they have on the causal effect test. Therefore, we observe an increasing pattern of p-values. When the p-value crosses the threshold of 0.05, the study conclusion would change qualitatively, from a significant finding to a non-significant one.

Specifically, when the unobserved confounder has a small positive association with the treatment ($\Gamma = 1.1$), the mortality difference between NTC and TC is highly significant, even if such a confounder has a large association with the outcome ($\Delta = 5$). When the association with treatment increases to $\Gamma = 2$, i.e., the odds of being admitted to the NTC may differ by a factor up to 2 in the matched pairs, such an imbalanced treatment assignment cannot nullify the underlying causal effect, except for the scenarios when the unobserved confounder has a large association with the outcome ($\Delta = 4$ or 5). If the associations between U and both admission and mortality are moderate, i.e., $\Gamma = 2$ and $\Delta = 2$, there is still strong evidence for a true causal effect ($p = 0.003$). But when the associations become larger, i.e., $\Gamma = 3$ and $\Delta = 3$, the evidence for a true causal effect is not as strong, since the p-value increases to 0.202. Since the sensitivity analysis computes the upper bound of the p-values for the causal effect test, it is somewhat conservative as it represents the worst-case scenario. Not knowing the unmeasured factor, it would be

TABLE 7.3

Upper Bound P-Values for Causal Effect Tests in Simultaneous Sensitivity Analysis

		Δ				
		1.1	2	3	4	5
	1.1	<0.001	<0.001	<0.001	<0.001	<0.001
	2	<0.001	0.003	0.022	0.060	0.108
Γ	3	<0.001	0.022	0.202	0.459	0.655
	4	<0.001	0.060	0.459	0.791	0.926
	5	<0.001	0.108	0.655	0.926	0.985

prudent not to rush to a decision and to request more scientific efforts to elucidate the causal relationship.

The calculation for the *p*-values is tedious in the conventional sensitivity analysis, as one has to redo the randomization test for every combination of sensitivity parameters and find the tipping point when the *p*-value crosses the threshold. The model-assisted approach simplifies the computation substantially by providing a closed-form solution of the sensitivity parameters leading to a non-significant causal effect test. Figure 7.4 plots the boundary curve of sensitivity parameters, where the upper-right area above the curve corresponds to non-significant tests and the lower-left area below the curve corresponds to significant tests. For example, the point (2, 2) is below the curve, which indicates, for $\Gamma = 2$ and $\Delta = 2$, that there is strong evidence for a true causal effect. The point (3, 3) is above the curve, which implies, $\Gamma = 3$ and $\Delta = 3$, there is not enough evidence for a causal effect. The asymptotes of the curve (the dashed lines) represent the scenario when either sensitivity parameter goes to infinity. The vertical asymptote is at $\Gamma = 1.48$, which implies, if the association between U and NTC admission is less than 1.48 (in odds ratio scale), there is always enough evidence for a true causal effect, regardless of how U correlates with death.

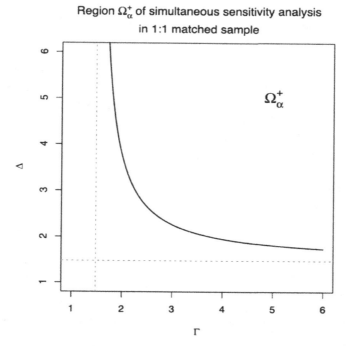

FIGURE 7.4
Contour Plot for Simultaneous Sensitivity Analysis.

Overall, the NEDS database provides strong evidence for mortality difference between NTCs and TCs, after adjusting for observed confounders through matching. Trauma patients are better off when being treated at TCs. This finding is moderately robust to hidden bias, as suggested by the sensitivity analysis. The causal effect test stays significant for small to medium values of sensitivity parameters, and it becomes non-significant for medium to large values. A more detailed analysis with both the pair-matched design and 1:3 matched design was presented in Nattino and Lu (2018) with R codes available as online supporting information (see https://onlinelibrary.wiley. com/doi/abs/10.1111/biom.12919).

In real-world data analysis, researchers do not have control over the treatment assignment mechanism. The causal effect estimation may suffer from biases arising from two sources. The overt bias can be handled with appropriate adjustment of observed covariates. The hidden bias presents a big challenge as no information is available on unobserved covariates. Without adequate treatment of unmeasured confounding, real-world data cannot support a strong argument for a causal relationship. Sensitivity analysis provides both a conceptual framework and a practical tool to assess how likely the finding based on observed data may change when the hidden bias is accounted for. It makes the RWE stronger and more defendable.

Acknowledgment

This work was partially supported by Grant 1R01 HS024263-01 from the Agency of Healthcare Research and Quality of the U.S. Department of Health and Human Services. The author thanks Giovanni Nattino, Junxin Shi, and Henry Xiang for the data set preparation, presentation of results, and insightful discussion on comparative trauma care research.

References

21st Century Cures Act 2016. https://www.congress.gov/114/plaws/publ255/PLAW-114publ255.pdf

Agency for Healthcare Research and Quality. 2016. Overview of the nationwide emergency department sample (NEDS). https://www.hcup-us.ahrq.gov/nedsoverview.jsp

Austin, P.C. 2014. The use of propensity score methods with survival or time-to-event outcomes: reporting measures of effect similar to those used in randomized experiments. *Statistics in Medicine*, 33(7), 1242–1258.

Bang, H., and Robins, J. M. 2005. Doubly robust estimation in missing data and causal inference models. *Biometrics*, 61, 962–972.

Belson, N.A. 2018. FDA's Historical Use of "Real World Evidence." Food and Drug Law Institute. https://www.fdli.org/2018/08/update-fdas-historical-use-of-real-world-evidence/

Centers for Disease Control and Prevention. 2006. History of the Surgeon General's Reports on Smoking and Health. https://www.cdc.gov/tobacco/data_statistics/sgr/history/index.htm

Cornfield, J., Haenszel, W., Hammond, E.C., Lilienfeld, A.M., Shimkin, M.B., and Wynder, E.L. 1959. Smoking and lung cancer: recent evidence and a discussion of some questions. *Journal of the National Cancer Institute*, 22, 173–203.

Ding, P. and VanderWeele, T. J. 2016. Sensitivity analysis without assumptions. *Epidemiology*. 27, 368–377.

Gastwirth, J.L., Krieger, A.M., and Rosenbaum, P.R. 1998. Dual and simultaneous sensitivity analysis for matched pairs. *Biometrika*, 85, 907–920.

Hansen, B.B. and Klopfer, S.O. 2006. Optimal full matching and related designs via network flows. *Journal of Computational and Graphical Statistics*, 15, 609–627.

Ho, D.E., Imai, K., King, G. and Stuart, E.A. 2007. Matching as nonparametric preprocessing for reducing model dependence in parametric causal inference. *Political Analysis*, 15, 199–236.

Imbens, G. W. 2003. Sensitivity to exogeneity assumptions in program evaluation. *The American Economic Review*, 93, 126–132.

Imbens, G.W. and Rubin, D.B. 2015. Causal inference: for statistics, *Social, and Biomedical Sciences, and introduction*. New York: Cambridge University Press.

Lin, D.Y., Psaty, B.M., and Kronmal, R.A. 1998. Assessing the sensitivity of regression results to unmeasured confounders in observational studies. *Biometrics*, 54, 948–963.

Lu B., Cai D., and Tong X. 2018.Testing causal effects in observational survival data using propensity score matching design. *Statistics in Medicine*, 37(11), 1846–1858.

Lu, B., Greevy, R., Xu, X., and Beck, C. 2011. Optimal nonbipartite matching and its statistical applications. *The American Statistician*, 65(1), 21–30.

Nattino G. and Lu B. 2018. Model assisted sensitivity analyses for hidden bias with binary outcomes." *Biometrics*, 74(4), 1141–1149.

Nattino, G., Lu, B., Shi, J., Lemeshow, S., and Xiang, H. 2020. Triplet Matching for Estimating Causal Effects with Three Treatment Arms: A Comparative Study of Mortality by Trauma Center Level, *the Journal of American Statistical Association*, published online April 2020, https://doi.org/10.1080/01621459.2020.1737078.

Neyman, J. 1990. On the Application of Probability Theory to Agricultural Experiments. Essay on Principles. Section 9 [Translated]. *Statistical Science*, 5(4), 465–472.

Robins, J.M., Hernan, M. A., and Brumback, B. 2000. Marginal structural models and causal inference in epidemiology. *Epidemiology*, 11, 550–560.

Robins, J.M., Rotnitzkey, A., and Scharfstein, D. 1999. Sensitivity analysis for selection bias and unmeasured confounding in missing data and causal inference models. In: E. Halloran and D. Berry, eds. *Statistical Models in Epidemiology*. New York: Springer, pp. 1–94.

Rosenbaum, P.R. 1991. A characterization of optimal designs for observational studies. *Journal of the Royal Statistical Society, Series B*, 53, 597–610.

Rosenbaum, P.R. 2002. *Observational Studies*. New York: Springer.

Rosenbaum, P.R. 2005. Sensitivity analysis in observational studies. In: B. S. Everitt and D. C. Howell, eds. *Encyclopedia of Statistics in Behavioral Science*. Chichester, UK: John Wiley & Sons; vol 4, pp. 1809–1814.

Rosenbaum, P.R. 2010. *Design of Observational Studies.* New York: Springer.

Rosenbaum, P.R. 2017. *Observation and Experiment: An Introduction to Causal Inference.* Cambridge, Massachusetts: Harvard University Press.

Rosenbaum, P.R. and Rubin, D.B. 1983a. The central role of the propensity score in observational studies for causal effects. *Biometrika,* 70, 41–55.

Rosenbaum P.R. and Rubin D. B. 1983b. Assessing sensitivity to an unobserved binary covariate in an observational study with binary outcome. *Journal of the Royal Statistical Society, Series B,* 45, 212–218.

Rubin, D.B. 1974. Estimating causal effects of treatments in randomized and nonrandomized studies. *Journal of Educational Psychology,* 66(5), 688–701.

Rubin, D.B. 2001. Using propensity scores to help design observational studies: application to the tobacco litigation. *Health Services & Outcomes Research Methodology,* 2, 169–188.

Shadish, W.R., Cook, T.D., and Campbell, D.T. 2002. *Experimental and Quasi-Experimental Designs for Generalized Causal Inference.* Boston: Houghton-Mifflin.

Shi, J., Lu, B., Wheeler, K.K., and Xiang, H. 2016. Unmeasured confounding in observational studies with multiple treatment arms. *Epidemiology,* 27, 624–632.

Stuart, E. 2010. Matching methods for causal inference: a review and a look forward. *Statistical Science,* 25(1), 1–21.

Tan, Z. 2007. Comment: Understanding OR, PS and DR. *Statistical Science,* 22(4), 560–568.

8

Introduction to Artificial Intelligence and Deep Learning with a Case Study in Analyzing Electronic Health Records for Drug Development

Xiaomao Li, Google, Qi Tang, Sanofi

8.1 Introduction to AI and Overview of Breakthroughs of AI in Drug Development

8.1.1 Why AI?

There have been three industrial revolutions in human history: the steam revolution characterized by steam-powered mechanical production and rail transportation; the electrification revolution represented by electric-powered mass production and assembly lines; and the information revolution led by the invention of computers and all kinds of electronics that facilitate information collection, storage, exchange, and data analytics (Schweb 2016). These industrial revolutions, particularly the third one, paved the way for the fourth industrial revolution, the digital revolution, which started with digitization and artificial intelligence (AI). We are currently in the fourth revolution, whether we believe it or not. Digitization enables the connection of different physical devices and collection and integration of various types of data measuring the whole world including the environment, our life, and our work (e.g., smart home and automated warehouse; Rajkumar et al. 2010). To gain insights from the big data collected through digitization and to make the devices smart, AI plays a central role (Dopico et al. 2016). If we make an analogy between the fourth industrial revolution and a human and if we say digitization is the left foot of a human, then AI is the right foot (Towers-Clark 2019). Recently, there has been a boom of AI exemplified by self-driving cars (Bojarski et al. 2016), cashier-less grocery stores (Polacco and Backes 2018), smart personal assistants that can make appointment phone calls for you (Haselton 2018), smart robots that can navigate complicated geographic areas and complete tasks autonomously (Nelson et al. 2019), and machines that can diagnose eye diseases without human intervention (Van Der Heijden et al. 2018).

8.1.2 What Is AI and How Do You Build an AI System?

The concept of AI was first created by the computer scientist Alan Turing, who envisioned AI as a machine that can think as a human (Li et al. 2018). The term AI was coined by another computer scientist, John McCarthy of MIT, who in 1965 defined AI as "the science and engineering of making intelligent machines" (Welsh 2019). A TED speaker once mentioned that a key factor to distinguishing AI versus other types of algorithms is that the "AI writes computer programs by itself." Of course, he did not mean that current AI is as smart as a human and can write these programs from the beginning to the end. What he meant was that an AI product will be able to decide on its own rules about how to engineer features from the inputs to achieve a goal. Using this definition, AI distinguishes itself from traditional machine learning methods, such as tree methods, expert systems, and almost all statistical methods, in which human hands coded the rules of how to extract features from inputs (Marr 2016). This unique feature makes AI more powerful than traditional machine learning methods and makes the interpretation of AI challenging.

The recent boom of AI began around the year 2010, when a huge data set of real-life images named ImageNet (Deng et al. 2009), which has more than 1000 classes of images and more than 14 million images with annotations by human, was used to evaluate the performance of computer vision algorithms. With ImageNet, different teams can compete to achieve higher accuracy on several visual recognition tasks. In 2015, the performance of the best algorithms surpassed the average human performance in image classification (He et al. 2015). Solving the problems of computer visions enables the machines to see and interpret the world, which fosters the boom of self-driving car technology, automated warehouses, cashier-less stores, and smart devices. The impact of the revolution in computer vision goes beyond this field. From the success of computer vision, people learned two things: first, the importance of big data, not just big in terms of size but also big in terms of varieties, and second, the central role of neural network algorithms in analyzing big data. With this knowledge, similar breakthroughs have been achieved in language translation (Young et al. 2018), text to speech with natural voices (Artemov et al. 2016), natural language processing, disease diagnosis using medical images (Esteva et al. 2017), and strategy games such as Go (Silver et al. 2016), Warcraft Dota 2 (Bansal et al. 2017), and StarCraft (Arulkumaran et al. 2019).

To build an AI system, there are three key components: data, algorithm, and computing power. Similar to other models, AI models may suffer from GIGO: garbage in and garbage out. An AI system is trained based on data fed into it and will make prediction and decisions based on the data it has learned from. If the data have bias, then the AI system built on it may be biased (Zou and Schiebinger 2018). An example of AI algorithm bias toward males is when it is asked to predict a person as a CEO. This bias occurs if it is trained on a set of real-life images of CEOs, since the majority of CEOs are male. Another example is that an AI-powered surveillance camera may fail to identify a violent shooting if the data fed into the algorithm has very few examples of mass shootings. Along with data, the next important component for building AI is the algorithm. Algorithms behind the aforementioned successes of AI are deep learning and reinforcement learning. Deep learning is a re-branded name of the neural network method, which was developed in the 1980s and has been a very popular method for AI since 2012 (LeCun et al. 2015). In the 2012 ImageNet competition in the field of computer vision, the best team is more than 40% better than the runner up and the algorithm used by the best team is a convolutional neural network (CNN) method (Krizhevsky et al. 2012; Alom et al. 2018). Suddenly, people within the computer vision field and other fields of the technology industry began to pay attention to this method. From then on, almost all teams participating in the ImageNet competition used CNN methods; the error rate kept decreasing and became even better than the average human level at the last ImageNet competition with an error rate of 2.25% (Hu et al. 2018). The success of deep learning methods in AI can be partially explained by neural science, because the architecture mimics how neurons interact with each other and how human brains work (Marblestone et al. 2016). Also, mathematically there is a universal approximation theorem proving that any bounded continuous relationship can be approximated by neural networks arbitrarily well (Csáji 2001). Along with data and the algorithm, the last component of AI is computing power. Many successful deep learning algorithms have millions to billions of parameters to be estimated based on a data set with millions of subjects. To complete the optimization procedure and obtain optimal estimate of the parameters within a reasonable amount of time, the central processing unit (CPU) itself is not sufficient enough. The graphic processing unit (GPU) and other types of chips designed specific for neural network optimization are needed to shorten the computer time from months to days (Chetlur et al. 2014; Abadi et al. 2016). The GPU was designed for fast computation to allow enhanced visual effects in computer games. It turns out that the optimization tasks for deep learning are very similar to those in computer graphics in that both involve addition and multiplication of large matrices, which can be processed through parallel computing by hundreds of cores in each GPU.

8.1.3 AI in Drug Development

After the success of AI in computer vision and strategy games, AI researchers and domain knowledge experts started to collaborate on the application of AI in drug development. The first identified area is drug discovery, where the volume of big data such as cellular images, cell line data and omics data keep increasing and challenge the traditional analytic methods (Chen et al. 2018). Since the first AI breakthroughs in computer vision, cellular images are the first among multiple modalities of data to be analyzed using

AI methods (Chen et al. 2016). Deep learning methods have been used to predict biologic properties of compounds based on single high-throughput imaging assays (Simm et al 2018), reducing the cost of drug development. Deep learning methods also have been used in image embeddings for drug repurposing (Victors, n.d.), which removes the noises caused by batch processing cellular images and enhances the signal for drug repurposing. Recently, DeepMind has developed a novel AI, AlphaFold, to predict 3D protein structures using genomic data (Evans et al. 2018). In 2018, they won first place in the 13th Critical Assessment of Structure Prediction (CASP) competition, which is an international protein folding prediction competition. Able to predict the 3D structure of proteins can play a fundamental role in drug discovery for diseases believed to be caused by misfolded proteins, such as Alzheimer's, Parkinson's, Huntington's, and cystic fibrosis (Evans et al. 2018).

Along with drug discovery, AI also makes inroads into clinical trials in the following areas: treatment compliance monitoring, prediction of patient outcomes in the real-world setting (Miotto et al. 2016), and prediction of clinical trial results (Artemov et al. 2016). Treatment compliance is a critical factor in the reduced treatment effect and increased burden on healthcare systems (Iuga and McGuire 2014). AI facial recognition technology together with smart phones was used to develop a medical assistant to assist patients taking oral treatments and increase treatment compliance. A small-scale study suggested that using such an AI platform can lead to a 50% increase of treatment compliance (Labovitz et al. 2017). However, there should be caution regarding improving compliance in a randomized clinical trial and whether it may lead to an increased placebo response, which may be a concern to be addressed in neuroscience studies. Along with monitoring and increasing treatment compliance, AI also has been used to predict patient outcomes in the real-world setting to assist physicians to better treat patients based on electronic health records (EHRs), which has abundant structured and unstructured health data of patients such as biomarker information, laboratory testing results, disease diagnosis, medication history, disease history, nurse notes, and physician notes. Because of the heterogeneous types of data to be modeled, AI plays a central role in EHR data integration and analytics (Bennett et al. 2012; Krittanawong et al. 2017; Mehta and Devarakonda 2018). For example, researchers were able to accurately predict medical outcomes of hospital patients such as, diagnosis, mortality, length of stay, and 30-day readmission, with accuracy ranging from 75% to 94% in terms of area under the curve (AUC) based on EHRs of 0.2 million patients with more than 46 billion data points (Rajkomar et al. 2018). Another example is that the AI method–based tumor tissue analysis leads to better prediction of patient 5-year disease-specific survival risks than human experts (Bychkov et al. 2018). However, the use of EHR and AI to predict patient outcome in clinical trials needs to be taken with caution because of potential population difference, confounding effects, missing data, and placebo effects, and the predictions may need to be adjusted before the study to inform clinical trial design and decision-making (Harrell and Lazzeroni 2018). In addition to predicting patient outcomes in the real-world setting, AI also has been applied to the prediction of clinical trial results based on deep learning analysis of transcriptomic data. Because of high failure rate in clinical trials, being able to predict which product is going to succeed in clinical trials can reduce the failure rate and the overall drug development costs. For example, transcriptomic data were used to predict side effects and drug-induced pathway activation, which is a surrogate for drug efficacy, based on deep learning methods. Then the results are fed into a classification model to estimate the probability of failure for a pharmaceutical product (Artemov et al. 2016). This two-stage approach delivered 83% cross-validation accuracy in predicting clinical trial results, and it was used to analyze the portfolios from multiple pharmaceutical companies.

8.2 A Minimalist Overview of Deep Learning Methods

Deep learning stands out as one of the most promising approaches for drug development. However, the literature on deep learning was primarily focused on key breakthroughs in computer vision, pattern recognition, and so forth. Its application in the medical field is less thoroughly surveyed. Despite several medical applications reported by the media, such as Google's application of deep learning on the detection of diabetic retinopathy (Gulshan et al. 2016), the major explorations of deep learning techniques for drug development remain undercovered.

Focusing on drug development, we will examine the promise of deep learning methodologies and figure out what it can add to the current practice by providing a new view of deep learning about from a biostatistical standpoint. We will also discuss what makes a successful application of deep learning when facing a task quite different from the traditional deep learning applications.

8.2.1 Why Deep Learning?

In the new era of technologies incorporated in the process of finding and experimenting with new treatments, there are many fundamental modeling issues to be solved. First, how do you accurately model the interaction between pharmacological treatment and the human body? It has always been difficult to come up with the correct parametric models based on pharmacological expertise due to the complexity of the biological mechanism in the human body. Second, how do you predict the benefit of a treatment to each individual patient? One-size-fits-all rarely exists in healthcare because patients are unique and their responses to a treatment can be heterogeneous. Last, how do you fully utilize totality of information from the big data generated in healthcare to inform drug development? Recently there has been rapid adoption of EHR systems, which make a large bulk of potentially unstructured observational data available to researchers. If modeled appropriately, the data offer the potential of enabling smarter decision-making in drug development.

Deep learning allows uncapped complexity of nonlinearity relationships and interactions between variables by concatenating, embedding, and joining the same units, e.g., nodes, layers, and networks. Such structural flexibility also opens the gate to modeling unstructured data together with structural data. In our example in Section 8.4, we will demonstrate how the medical history and physician notes can be incorporated into the modeling without feature engineering.

With the growing need for personalized medications, the traditional parametric modeling framework struggles to identify heterogeneous treatment effects with only limited amounts of patient data collected being used in the modeling process. This is due to the limitation of parametric models in which the interaction between variables and their functional form have to be explicitly set up. In contrast, deep learning can extract information from the millions or billions of data points because of the model complexity.

8.2.2 What Is Deep Learning?

Deep learning is a re-branded name of an old class of methods, named neural networks, with new engineering tricks making the optimization of the networks faster and better. Neural networks are networks of artificial neurons mimicking how the human brain functions, where information is transmitted from one neuron to multiple other neurons after being processed in that neuron. The transmission process is one way. Figure 8.1 displays a simple feed-forward neural network with only one hidden layer. The predictors, x_1 and x_2, are fed into the input layer where each neuron represents one input

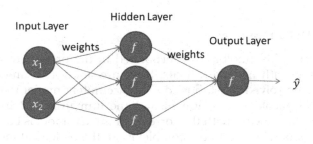

FIGURE 8.1
Illustration of a simple one hidden layer neural network.

variable. Then the data flow into the hidden layer in a weighted fashion and get transformed by a function *f*, called the activation function, which transforms the weighted input into an output. The output from each neuron in the hidden layer then flows into the output layer in a weighted fashion and, after being transformed by the activation function *f*, the response variable is predicted as $\hat{y}$. Usually the function *f* is a nonlinear function of the weighted sum of the inputs. If *f* is a linear function, the hidden layer is redundant and the neural network becomes a linear regression model. With more hidden layers, deep learning has the potential of modeling complicated interactions and nonlinear relationships between inputs and outputs.

The design of deep learning breaks apart from the traditional modeling thinking pattern in the sense that the model can easily have more parameters than the number of samples, which may lead to an overfitting issue if not regularized appropriately. The optimization of deep learning models relies on several recently developed techniques. An advantage of having more parameters is be able to do feature engineering automatically by deep learning models without human intervention as long as the relationship between input and output is a smooth bounded function. This is quite different from the traditional parametric models, for which hand engineering is often conducted before feeding the hand-engineered data into a model, for example, log transformation.

To build a feed-forward neural network, five key elements of the neural network need to be specified: (1) the variables fed into the input layer, (2) the number of neurons in each layer, (3) the activation function, (4) the number of layers, and (5) the response variable to be predicted in the output layer. These five elements are illustrated in Figure 8.2.

Figure 8.3 visualizes six commonly used activation functions. One often needs to compare the performance of different activation functions to choose the optimal one for each problem.

8.2.3 What Makes a Good Deep Learning Application?

The engineering flexibility of the deep learning framework and the accessibility of platforms, e.g., Tensorflow and Pytorch, make a thriving deep learning community. From both academia and industries, there are various types of deep learning applications succeeding in their specialized areas, including convolutional neural network (CNN), recurrent neural network (RNN), Long short-term memory (LTSM), and many others. In fact, for beginners, choosing the right type of neural network has become troublesome, not to mention tuning the structure and hyperparameters, which are critical for the ultimate performance. In this section, we list several key points that we think are important for deep learning applications.

First, an excellent deep learning framework always has a special design that suits the application. CNN enjoys an unmatched performance on image recognition, RNN succeeds in natural language processing, and LTSM

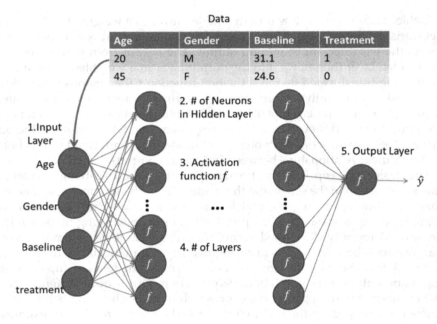

FIGURE 8.2
Five key elements of a feed forward neural network.

dominates time series modeling for a period of time. Behind the successes of these methods are their intuitive designs, which utilize the structure of the data. We will introduce our study in detail in Section 8.4. We chose a modified CNN as it suits the repeated measurements of patients and reflects the trajectory of patients' disease progressions.

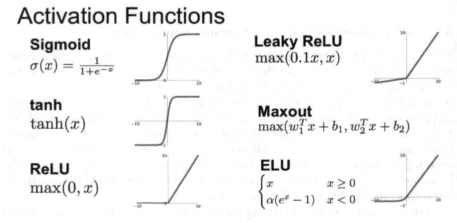

FIGURE 8.3
Six commonly used activation functions.

Second, a good application usually comes with a balance between model complexity and fitting power. The neural network model that is deep and wide enough has the potential to model an unlimited amount of complexities between predictors and outcomes. However, whether such a complicated model can converge into a stable solution within a certain period of time and with a certain number of observations is not necessarily an easy question to answer. In addition, an overcomplicated model leads to overfitting or brings trouble for hyperparameter tuning. A veteran deep learning modeler does not always go for the deepest or most complicated structure, usually they settle with what suits the application. In our study, we eventually chose a CNN, which is not the deepest, after considering the noisy nature of the data set and the computational resources available to us.

Third, a reliable hyperparameter tuning framework is often an essential part of a good deep learning application. Parameter tuning is the key component of the neural network, which is critical for finding the balance point between overfitting and underfitting. An overly complicated tuning framework can bring extensive burden to the system and hinder the progress of the application. In our study, we made most of the parameters default and only tune the dropout rate and L2 penalty through grid search. Our results indicate that the amount of tuning is enough to exploit the potential of the CNN model.

8.3 Introduction of the Big Data in Clinical Space: EHR

8.3.1 Challenges of Analyzing EHR

Despite the demonstrated potential of EHR data sets, there are still challenges to fully utilize their rich information. The difficulties come from the observational nature of the EHR data set and the usually complex process of data collection. Various issues can be categorized into three types, i.e., the messiness of the data, missingness, and confounding issues.

Compared with experimental data that are usually collected under a rigorous schema, EHR data sets are generally more error prone. Among many factors that contribute to the reality, the lack of coordination is probably the most prominent. EHR data sets are usually collected for purposes not related to research. They often go through several agents until being finally consumed by a research institution. The impossibility of quality control and information sharing between end users and data collectors created the most difficulties. Measurements are sometimes recorded with different units, or the same units but wrongly located decimal separators. Also, there are misspelled medications, inconsistent styles of capitalization and abbreviation, and prescriptions that are phased differently.

EHR data sets often suffer from severe missingness, and even high data quality does not rule out missingness. For example, because physicians prescribe examinations according to the conditions of the patients, it is natural that many measurements will be missing for most of the patients. For those who had a certain measurement, it is not guaranteed that this measurement will continue to be updated through the life course of the patient. Consequently, usually about 90% of the measurements are missing for all patient quarters. We will tackle this harsh situation in Section 8.4.

Confounding issues in EHR data sets are easily overlooked. In fact, this might actually cause the most severe flaws for any causal studies. Physicians give prescriptions according to the condition of patients, creating a natural confounding that the prescriptions received by the patients are partially determined by the status of the patients, which usually lead to an amplified treatment effect. In Section 8.3, we present a strategy to incorporate as much information as possible so that the confounding issue can be alleviated.

8.4 A Case Study Using Deep Learning to Analyze EHR

To demonstrate the application of deep learning techniques for drug development, we present a study of diabetic patients' responses to SGLT-2 inhibitors using an EHR data set. The purpose of this study is to identify subpopulations with effect heterogeneities of SGLT-2 inhibitors. The knowledge of such subpopulations has two subsequent benefits. First, future drug development can target these newly discovered subpopulations who do not have enough response to the existing therapies. Second, the pharmaceutical company may adjust the marketing strategies of drugs emphasizing extraordinary effects on specific subpopulations.

The data set used is a high-quality EHR data set with 4 million patients and 254 million visits in total. It also contains 0.3 million types of medications and other information including operation, medical history, complaints, lab tests, and diagnosis.

Rich content, tremendous opportunities, and unseen challenges are presented with this data set. Along with all the difficulties brought by the pure size of the data, how to utilize the raw and unstructured data seems an even harder question. Diagnosis information might not be recorded due to the missingness of the ICD-9/ICD-10 code. Medications are not perfectly categorized due to rxnorm missing or they are simply hard to classify. There are large percentages of missing entries in longitudinal data, especially for medical history. Typos and wrong units also impose great threats by increasing the number of outliers. In addition, there are unclassified observations and physician notes that are impossible for manual coding considering the size of the data.

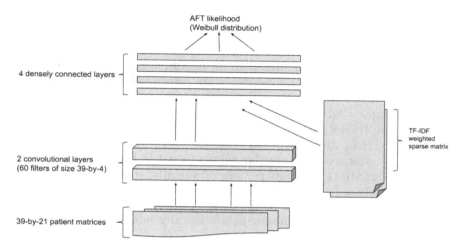

FIGURE 8.4
The proposed CNN with patient matrices and term frequency–inverse document frequency (TF-IDF) weighted texts.

In this section, we will demonstrate how these challenges are tackled by a properly designed CNN with extra features, as in Figure 8.4. Then we examine the effectiveness of the designed CNNs by their abilities to predict two outcome variables, a continuous endpoint, body mass index (BMI), and a survival endpoint, cardiovascular event. With a CNN that best predicts the outcome, we subsequently adopted the virtual twin strategy to identify the subpopulations.

8.4.1 Alignment of Diabetic Patients

Due to the volume of the EHR data set and the presence of repeated measures at different periods of patients with distinct health conditions and disease progressions, additional alignment is done to alleviate the confounding issue. The alignment model we used here is a propensity score model derived from a previous study based on the same data set. Patients who had metformin prescriptions are selected into the treatment group given certain conditions, whereas the remaining patients are selected for the control group if their propensities fall into the same strata.

It should be noted that the extra alignment at the cost of a smaller sample size is not generally necessary. In this study, it serves as a precautionary strategy in case of the violation of ignorability assumption, which, in fact, is unlikely to be true given the number of measures that are included in this study.

8.4.2 Convolutional Layers for EHR Data

The CNNs proposed in this section are designed using a two-step approach. First, the convolutional layers are designed based on the structure of the

EHR. Subsequently, the output layer is specially designed for each outcome variable. The number of layers is essentially a hyperparameter that is determined by the performance of the final models.

The EHR data set is organized in an event-based structure. For each visit of a patient, only several measures are recorded based on the activity of the visit. A set of 39 predictors are manually coded, including demographics, historic lab tests (hemoglobin [Hb]A1c, estimated glomerular filtration rate [EGFR], BMI, low-density lipoprotein [LDL], high-density lipoprotein [HDL], diastolic blood pressure [DBP], systolic blood pressure [SBP]), and historic cardiovascular events (heart failure, coronary artery disease, myocardial infarction, peripheral vascular disease). The selection of these variables is mainly justified by previous studies based on the same data set. For each predictor, there could be 29 quarterly repeated measures, although these measures are usually missing for most of the quarters.

Consequently, we have a 2D matrix for each patient with the X-dimension length of 21 representing the quarters and the Y-dimension length of 39 holding the value of the predictors.

This 21×39 matrix can be treated as an image in the image recognition settings. Our CNN contains 2 convolutional layers with 60 filters of size 4×39 for each layer because the trajectory of the quarterly measures for each predictor matters, but the order of the predictors does not. The stride size is set to 1 quarter. The max-pooling after the filtering has a stride size of two quarters. There are four fully connected layers following the convolutional layers with 200 neurons per layer. The dropout rate is 0.5. The complete structure of the proposed CNN is depicted in Figure 8.4.

Due to the size of this data set and the scope of this study, the parameters and network structures are decided based on experience. We have no doubt that further hyperparameter tuning will increase the performance of the model.

8.4.3 Text Information from Unstructured Data

To fully utilize the treasures in this data set, one cannot overlook the unstructured data. We make one step further toward complete utilization by combining text analysis with the CNN. From the uncategorized observations and physician notes, we extract the top 1000 medical keywords and calculate their TF-IDF weights for each patient. According to the (formula), Keywords that presented in a few documents for many times each will have larger weights while those presented in many documents for a few times each will have smaller weights. As a result, we have one 1000 vector length for the total weights of all keywords associated with each patient. These weight vectors are then fully connected to the first dense layer from which they will interact with the outputs of convolutional layers.

8.4.4 Missing Data Imputation

In the previous sections, we explained how the matrices of patients' measurements are used to construct the CNN. A matrix constitutes a valid input for the CNN only if the missing entries of the matrices are properly handled. In addition to the several missing mechanisms that we mentioned in Section 8.4, the construction of matrices will result in more missing values, because repeated measurements at all periods are required for all the time-varying measurements. In our case, there are often patients with more than 50% missing entries for which we have to meticulously choose the strategy to handle the missing data.

There are several strategies for handling missing data including forward/backward filling, multiple imputations, discretizing, and matrix completion. We will discuss these strategies briefly in this section,

Forward and backward fillings are common approaches for missing data when dealing with time series or longitudinal data. Forward filling takes the last observation and uses it to fill any subsequent missing entries. Similarly, backward filling always searches for the next observation to fill a missing entry. Their advantages lie in simplicity since they do involve any forms of modeling and thus can be executed with great efficiency. The drawback of such imputation strategies is that they are unable to share information across variables as all the fillings are done separately for each variable. Also, in our case, some patients have sparsely observed measures so that their two measures of a certain type can be separated by months or even years of missing. In such a situation, it is hard to believe that the forward/backward filling is still a good strategy.

Multiple imputation is a very popular statistical modeling approach in medical research. Statistical models are designed for each variable with missingness, usually using the observed entries of the variable as the outcome and other variables are covariates. Under the assumption of missing at random (MAR), this strategy relies on the information from the observed population to impute the unobserved population. The fact that there are multiple variables with missingness leads to the practice of multiple imputation where multiply imputed data sets are generated to counter the variation from random starting points. All the subsequent modeling needs to be replicated on all the data sets and their results need to be summarized. We chose not to use multiple imputation because every single run of CNN takes hours, which makes it impossible to replicate the results on hundreds of data sets.

Matrix completion is a concept in machine learning and signal processing. Originally designed to recover a sparsely measured matrix, the algorithm fills up the missing entries in a way that the resulting matrix will have the lowest rank in all possible choices. Mathematically, the lowest rank usually means the highest order, i.e., the matrix contains most information from the interaction of variables. There are studies showing that this approach can be used for missing data imputation when the missingness is MAR (e.g., Ma

& Chen 2019, Sportisse 2020). Computationally, this approach can be solved using convex optimization programs. In our study, we chose to use matrix imputation because of its computational efficiency and its ability to recover a matrix with potentially only 1% of the observed entries, which suits our needs in dealing with a large number of patients with sparse measurements.

8.4.5 Continuous Endpoints: HbA1c, BMI

As diabetic patients often suffer from obesity, BMI has been a very important index for measuring diabetes progression. To evaluate the validity of the proposed network structure, we examine its ability to predict the BMI given the predictors.

Although it is a typical regression problem, predicting BMI is intrinsically not easy because of the amount of missingness in this data set and the noisy nature of EHR data. Therefore, several methods are included for comparison, including ordinary least-squares (OLS) regression, randomForest, a simple deep neural network (DNN) approach, and the proposed CNN with TF-IDF weighted text. The OLS and the randomForest are the typical regression methods used in statistics and machine learning communities. Limited by the scope of this study, we do not cover the details of these methods. The simple DNN method shares the same set of predictors with quarterly repeated measures. The only difference is that the DNN does not impose any convolutional layers on the data; rather, it uses a flattened vector of length 819 (21 × 39) as the input layer. There are 10 fully connected layers with 400 neurons for each layer. The dropout rate is the same as the CNN approach. Table 8.1 shows the performance of these methods in terms of R-square based on fivefold cross-validation.

Table 8.1 proved the difficulty of predicting BMI for diabetic patients. All methods have R-squares around 0.5. The classic DNN does not beat the randomForest, which is extremely robust in noisy settings. However, the proposed CNN approach actually enjoys a 2% improvement, which implies the trajectories of predictors' values contribute to the prediction aside from the values themselves. In addition, adding text information can get a further edge of 1%. This verified the hypothesis that the text contains extra information

TABLE 8.1

R-Squares of Various Methods

Methods	R^2
OLS	0.46
Random Forest	0.51
Deep Neural Network	0.51
Convolutional Neural Network	0.53
CNN with TF-IDF weighted Text	0.54

about the patients, but this marginal improvement can hardly justify the increased training time and the complexity of the model.

8.4.6 Survival Endpoint: MACE

We solve the parameter optimization using back-propagation, which theoretically can work for any combination of differentiable loss functions. Moving from the continuous endpoint to survival endpoint is not very difficult. The structure of the network does not need any modification except the output layer changes from least-square loss to survival loss. Here we choose the accelerated failure time (AFT) model over the Cox model as the latter only uses observations without events, which is only 4.47% of the whole population. To simplify the problem, we assume that the event time follows a Weibull distribution. In the output layer of the CNN model, the loss function is the log-likelihood of a Weibull distribution with fixed $k = 2$ and λ being the linear combination of all the neurons in the output layer.

Similar to the previous section, there are linear AFT models, DNNs, CNNs, and CNNs with text information in the comparison. Randomforest is left out because it is not straightforward enough to adapt tree-based methods for survival analysis. Table 8.2 shows the performance in terms of AUC, concordance, and concordance on patients with cardiovascular events. To give a reference, the famous Framingham Risk Score only has a concordance of 0.69. Several conclusions can be drawn from the table. First, it is relatively easy to tell cardiovascular patients from non-cardiovascular patients. Second, it is more difficult to tell high-risk cardiovascular patients from low-risk cardiovascular patients. Finally, DNN/CNNs provide a more accurate prediction of whether a patient will have events by a specific time.

8.4.7 Virtual Twin Method

In the previous sections, we demonstrated how a powerful machine learning framework can be constructed to predict multiple endpoints. Such a framework is itself of great importance and it helps physicians to evaluate the disease progression of new patients. However, its connection with drug

TABLE 8.2

R-Squares of Various Methods

Methods	Concordance	Concordance on CV	Average AUC
Linear Cox model	0.73	0.49	0.67
DNN + AFT	0.76	0.49	0.75
CNN + AFT	0.76	0.52	0.77
CNN + AFT + text	0.77	0.54	0.78

development is less exposed. In this section, we present our solution using the virtual twin method.

Causal inference on observational data has always been challenging, especially when the data set involves extended periods, multiple sources, and potentially different scopes for data collection. However, this is the case of most EHR data sets. Therefore, we need a rigorous design so that we can avoid drawing conclusions based on spurious correlations. The framework used in this study allows us to discuss the causality of the medications and outcomes because of two features. First, the CNN model possess the ability to approximate any forms of interactions between the treatments and patients' medical conditions. Thus, it captures heterogeneities much better compared with the traditional parameter models where choosing functional form plays an overly important role in whether the model is mis-specified or not. Second, the EHR data set contains rich content of the patients and the neural network makes use of them by incorporating raw text information into the modeling. Consequently, it is generally safer to say that certain key assumptions, like ignorability assumption 1, that we are going to make in this study are more likely to hold.

Based on the fitted model, we can estimate the individual treatment effect for a certain patient by plugging in two patient matrices with the only difference being the medication record. Then the corresponding difference between the outcomes constitutes an estimate of the effect of changing medications from one to another. In this study, this interpretation relies on the ignorability assumption, which is believed to hold given the amount of information collected for each patient. Figure 8.5 shows the logic of this procedure.

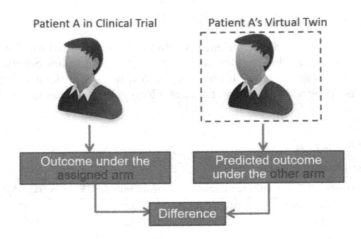

FIGURE 8.5
Virtual twin for individual treatment effect.

Note that the individual treatment effect should not be interpreted as a reliable indication of what would have happened assuming the patient took another type of medication. Although the bias is controlled, there is still a chance that our estimate has a high variance due to the noisy nature of the EHR data set. Nonetheless, the estimated individual treatment effects can be used collectively, for example, one can estimate the average treatment effect (ATE) by averaging over individual treatment effects (ITEs) of all individuals, or one can estimate the ATE for a subpopulation. The tree-based methods can serve for the latter by automatically identifying the subpopulations in which the ATE is significantly higher or lower than the overall ATE for the population.

Using the virtual twin framework on the EHR data set, we study the effect of using metformin medication versus non-metformin medications, which involves, first, estimating the individual treatment effect estimated from customized CNN and, second, using the regression tree to identify the subgroups. From the pool of patients, we did learn some suggestive subgroups with effect heterogeneities, part of which are summarized in Figure 8.6. It can be inferred from the tree structure that most of the splits are associated with either demographical information, such as age, or important measurements, such as LDL, HDL, or BMI. Not surprisingly, these patterns require further verification to be used in practices.

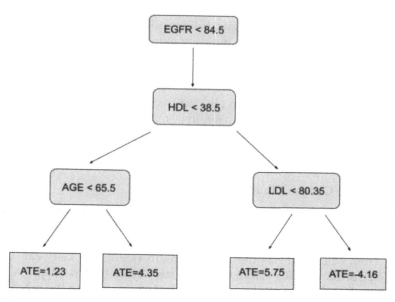

FIGURE 8.6
Partial tree structure of effect heterogeneity.

8.5 Introduction to Cloud Computing

In this section, we will briefly discuss the infrastructure for deep learning applications. Decisions concerning the infrastructure should always be made according to the target use case and the budget available.

8.5.1 Why Cloud Computing?

What makes a market worth $200 billion? According to GartnerForecasts (2018), this number will grow to 400 billion by 2020 with Software as a Service (SaaS) and Infrastructure as a Service (IaaS) to Platform as a Service (PaaS) summing up together. The rapid adoptions are backed up by several unique advantages of cloud service that cannot be replaced by traditional computational platforms.

Moving to the cloud is first considered as a cost-saving strategy. Small businesses are usually unable to invest and maintain a large infrastructure with cutting-edge technologies. Moving to the cloud is a capital expenditure–free and operational agile choice that is especially beneficial to smaller companies who put great value in their cash flow. When a business has not yet become the focus of the company, it is always better to try it out on the cloud so that it can be scaled up or scaled down according to the market feedback.

Cloud platforms can boost collaboration and innovation within a company. It is likely to increase productivity when multiple teams can access, edit, and share documents anytime and from anywhere. Cloud-based workflow, file sharing, and document control give full visibility of the collaborations. More importantly, cloud providers are building more of their services on the cloud, such as machine learning application and open-source software, so that teams with common interests in exploring the most advanced technologies can share their findings easily.

Furthermore, a cloud platform also can reduce the maintenance effort by providing services such as security, disaster recovery, automatic software updates, and system monitoring. Together they can reduce a large amount of IT cost.

8.5.2 How to Choose Cloud?

There are mainly three cloud service providers that together had most of the market share and growth. Amazon Web Services (AWS) from Amazon has been the first player in this field and occupied close to 40% of the market. Azure from Microsoft has the fastest growth rate in the last year. Google Cloud Performance (GCP) from Google is usually viewed as a big challenger even though their current performance is not comparable to the other two.

It is now well accepted that AWS has become the clear leader in the market. The pace of their innovations and new feature launches has not been matched by any other companies. Their cloud services are cheap to try and easy to set up. The pure scale of AWS' user base brings more data, which can be used to improve the services and larger revenue to expand the team. The thriving ecosystem eventually makes AWS the default choice to whoever wants to try out a cloud service.

Azure, on the other hand, has focused on specific use cases and has some advantages over AWS in some fields. For example, it is believed that their support to the .Net Framework and SQL database is beyond what AWS can achieve at this point. In addition, Microsoft successfully leveraged its experience working with enterprise users to make Azure more attractive. The Office ecosystem is unarguably one good reason for companies to choose Azure over AWS. Azure also leads in hybrid cloud service, which is a key factor for companies not willing to upload all their data on the cloud and thus need the bridge between private cloud and public cloud.

GCP has never been excluded in similar comparisons partially due to the high media exposure of Google and its parent company Alphabet. Similar to Azure, GCP also has been trying to secure a proportion of the market using its own advantage, i.e., Google's leading position in machine learning and AI. It is claimed that GCP provides better services than AWS and Azure when it comes to image recognition, voice assistance, and data-based applications. It is predicted that GCP is likely to solidify its third position in the market in the long run. It is worth mentioning that GCP has a large number of personal users due to better support for personal accounts and its association with open-source machine learning platforms, like TensorFlow.

Our application runs on an AWS EC2 instance (p3.16xlarge) that has 8 GPUs. For larger deep learning applications, it is essential to choose instances with multiple GPUs so that training time will not be too much of an obstacle for exploring network structures and parameter tuning. In contrast, for smaller deep learning applications, an instance with a single GCU can reduce cost as well as the code complexity.

References

Abadi, M., Barham, P., Chen, J., Chen, Z., Davis, A., Dean, J., Devin, M., Ghemawat, S., Irving, G., Isard, M., et al. 2016. Tensorflow: a system for large-scale machine learning. In 12th {USENIX} Symposium on Operating Systems Design and Implementation ({OSDI} 16), 265–283.

Alom, M.Z., Taha, T.M., Yakopcic, C., Westberg, S., Sidike, P., Nasrin, M.S., Van Esesn, B.C., Awwal, A. A. S. and Asari, V. K. 2018. The history began from AlexNet: a comprehensive survey on deep learning approaches. *arXiv preprint arXiv:1803.01164*.

Artemov, A.V., Putin, E., Vanhaelen, Q., Aliper, A., Ozerov, I.V., and Zhavoronkov, A. 2016. Integrated deep learned transcriptomic and structure based predictor of clinical trials outcomes. *bioRxiv*, p. 095653.

Arulkumaran, K., Cully, A., and Togelius, J. 2019. Alphastar: an evolutionary computation perspective. *arXiv preprint arXiv:1902.01724*.

Bansal, T., Pachocki, J., Sidor, S., Sutskever, I., and Mordatch, I. 2017. Emergent complexity via multi-agent competition. *arXiv preprint arXiv:1710.03748*.

Bennett, C.C., Doub, T.W., and Selove, R. 2012. EHRs connect research and practice: where predictive modeling, artificial intelligence, and clinical decision support intersect. *Health Policy and Technology*, 1(2), 105–114.

Bojarski, M., Del Testa, D., Dworakowski, D., Firner, B., Flepp, B., Goyal, P., Jackel, L.D., Monfort, M., Muller, U., Zhang, J., et al. 2016. End to end learning for self-driving cars. *arXiv preprint arXiv:1604.07316*.

Bychkov, D., Linder, N., Turkki, R., Nordling, S., Kovanen, P. E., Verrill, C., Walliander, M., Lundin, M., Haglund, C., and Lundin, J. 2018. Deep learning based tissue analysis predicts outcome in colorectal cancer. *Scientific Reports*, 8(1), 3395.

Chen, C.L., Mahjoubfar, A., Tai, L.-C., Blaby, I.K., Huang, A., Niazi, K.R., and Jalali, B. 2016. Deep learning in label-free cell classification. *Scientific Reports*, 6, 21471.

Chen, H., Engkvist, O., Wang, Y., Olivecrona, M., and Blaschke, T. 2018. The rise of deep learning in drug discovery. *Drug Discovery Today*, 23(6), 1241–1250.

Chetlur, S., Woolley, C., Vandermersch, P., Cohen, J., Tran, J., Catanzaro, B., and Shelhamer, E. 2014. cuDNN: efficient primitives for deep learning. *arXiv preprint arXiv:1410.0759*.

Csáji, B.C. 2001. Approximation with artificial neural networks. *Faculty of Sciences, Etvs Lor60d University, Hungary*, 24, 48.

Deng, J., Dong, W., Socher, R., Li, L.-J., Li, K., and Fei-Fei, L. 2009. Imagenet: a large-scale hierarchical image database. In 2009 IEEE Conference on Computer Vision and Pattern Recognition, IEEE, pp. 248–255.

Dopico, M., Gomez, A., De la Fuente, D., García, N., Rosillo, R., and Puche, J. 2016. A vision of industry 4.0 from an artificial intelligence point of view. In Proceedings on the International Conference on Artificial Intelligence (ICAI), 407.

Esteva, A., Kuprel, B., Novoa, R.A., Ko, J., Swetter, S.M., Blau, H.M., and Thrun, S. 2017. Dermatologist-level classification of skin cancer with deep neural networks. *Nature*, 542(7639), 115.

Evans, R., Jumper, J., Kirkpatrick, J., Sifre, L., Green, T., Qin, C., Zidek, A., Nelson, A., Bridgland, A., Penedones, H., et al. 2018. De novo structure prediction with deeplearning based scoring. *Annual Review of Biochemistry*, 77, 363–382.

GartnerForecasts. 2018. Gartner forecasts worldwide public cloud revenue to grow 17.3 percent in 2019. https://www.gartner.com/en/newsroom/press-releases /2018-09-12-gartner-forecasts-worldwide-public-cloud-revenue-to-grow-17-percent-in-2019

Gulshan, V., Peng, L., Coram, M., Stumpe, M C., Wu, D., Narayanaswamy, A., Venugopalan, S., Widner, K., Madams, T., Cuadros, J., et al. 2016. Development and validation of a deep learning algorithm for detection of diabetic retinopathy in retinal fundus photographs. *JAMA*, 316(22), 2402–2410.

Harrell, F. and Lazzeroni, L. 2018. EHRS and RCTS: outcome prediction vs. optimal treatment selection. https://www.fharrell.com/post/ehrs-rcts/

Haselton, T. 2018. Google's assistant is getting so smart it can place phone calls and humans think it's real. https://www.cnbc.com/2018/05/08/googles-assistant-will-soon-place-phone-calls-to-book-appointments.html

He, K., Zhang, X., Ren, S., and Sun, J. 2015. Delving deep into rectifiers: surpassing human-level performance on Imagenet classification. In Proceedings of the IEEE International Conference on Computer Vision, pp. 1026–1034.

Hu, J., Shen, L., and Sun, G. 2018. Squeeze-and-excitation networks. In Proceedings of the IEEE Conference on Computer Vision and Pattern Recognition, 7132–7141.

Iuga, A.O. and McGuire, M.J. 2014. Adherence and health care costs. *Risk Management and Healthcare Policy*, 7, 35.

Krittanawong, C., Zhang, H., Wang, Z., Aydar, M., and Kitai, T. 2017. Artificial intelligence in precision cardiovascular medicine. *Journal of the American College of Cardiology*, 69(21), 2657–2664.

Krizhevsky, A., Sutskever, I., and Hinton, G.E. 2012. ImageNet classification with deep convolutional neural networks. *Advances in Neural Information Processing Systems*, 1097–1105.

Labovitz, D.L., Shafner, L., Reyes Gil, M., Virmani, D., and Hanina, A. 2017. Using artificial intelligence to reduce the risk of nonadherence in patients on anticoagulation therapy. *Stroke*, 48(5), 1416–1419.

LeCun, Y., Bengio, Y., and Hinton, G. 2015. Deep learning. *Nature*, 521(7553), 436.

Li, L., Zheng, N.-N., and Wang, F.-Y. 2018. On the crossroad of artificial intelligence: a revisit to Alan Turing and Norbert Wiener. *IEEE Transactions on Cybernetics*, 49(10), 3618–3626.

Ma, W., & Chen, G. H. (2019). Missing Not at Random in Matrix Completion: The Effectiveness of Estimating Missingness Probabilities Under a Low Nuclear Norm Assumption. *In Advances in 33rd Neural Information Processing Systems*, 14900–14909.

Marblestone, A.H., Wayne, G., and Kording, K.P. 2016. Toward an integration of deep learning and neuroscience. *Frontiers in Computational Neuroscience*, 10, 94.

Marr, B. 2016. What is the difference between deep learning, machine learning and AI? https://www.forbes.com/sites/bernardmarr/2016/12/08/what-is-the-difference-between-deep-learning-machine-learning-and-ai/6c3ea33726cf

Mehta, N. and Devarakonda, M.V. 2018. Machine learning, natural language programming, and electronic health records: The next step in the artificial intelligence journey? *Journal of Allergy and Clinical Immunology*, 141(6), 2019–2021.

Miotto, R., Li, L., Kidd, B.A., and Dudley, J.T. 2016. Deep patient: an unsupervised representation to predict the future of patients from the electronic health records. *Scientific Reports* 6, 26094.

Nelson, G., Saunders, A., and Playter, R. 2019. The PETMAN and Atlas robots at Boston Dynamics. *Humanoid Robotics: A Reference*, 169–186.

Polacco, A. and Backes, K. 2018. The Amazon Go concept: implications, applications, and sustainability. *Journal of Business & Management*, 24(1).

Rajkomar, A., Oren, E., Chen, K., Dai, A.M., Hajaj, N., Hardt, M., Liu, P.J., Liu, X., Marcus, J., Sun, M., et al. 2018. Scalable and accurate deep learning with electronic health records. *NPJ Digital Medicine*, 1(1), 18.

Rajkumar, R., Lee, I., Sha, L., and Stankovic, J. 2010. Cyber-physical systems: the next computing revolution. *In Design Automation Conference, IEEE*, 731–736.

Schweb, K. 2016. The fourth industrial revolution: what it means, how to respond. https://www.weforum.org/agenda/2016/01/the-fourth-industrialrevolution-what-it-means-and-how-to-respond/

Silver, D., Huang, A., Maddison, C.J., Guez, A., Sifre, L., Van Den Driessche, G., Schrittwieser, J., Antonoglou, I., Panneershelvam, V., Lanctot, M., et al. 2016. Mastering the game of go with deep neural networks and tree search. *Nature*, 529(7587), 484.

Simm, J., Klambauer, G., Arany, A., Steijaert, M., Wegner, J.K., Gustin, E., Chupakhin, V., Chong, Y.T., Vialard, J., Buijnsters, P., et al. 2018. Repurposing high-throughput image assays enables biological activity prediction for drug discovery. *Cell Chemical Biology*, 25(5), 611–618.

Sportisse, A., Boyer, C., & Josse, J. (2020). Imputation and low-rank estimation with Missing Not At Random data. *Statistics and Computing*, 30(6), 1629–1643.

Towers-Clark, C. 2019. Big data, IoT and AI, part one: Three sides of the same coin. https://www.forbes.com/sites/charlestowersclark/2019/02/15/big-data-iot-and-ai-part-one-three-sides-of-the-same-coin/#ab8281969da6

Van Der Heijden, A.A., Abramoff, M.D., Verbraak, F., van Hecke, M.V., Liem, A., and Nijpels, G. 2018. Validation of automated screening for referable diabetic retinopathy with the IDX-DR device in the Hoorn diabetes care system. *Acta Ophthalmologica*, 96(1), 63–68.

Victors, M. n.d. Robust deep image embeddings for drug repurposing - Mason Victors, ReWork Health. https://www.youtube.com/watch?v=mkKIxQMHMy8

Welsh, R. 2019. Defining artificial intelligence. *SMPTE Motion Imaging Journal*, 128(1), 26–32.

Young, T., Hazarika, D., Poria, S., and Cambria, E. 2018. Recent trends in deep learning based natural language processing. *IEEE Computational Intelligence Magazine*, 13(3), 55–75.

Zou, J. and Schiebinger, L. 2018. AI can be sexist and racist—it's time to make it fair. *Nature*, 559(7714), 324–326.

Index

Note: Locators in *italics* represent figures and **bold** indicate tables in the text.

A

Academy of Managed Care Pharmacy (AMCP), 119
Accelerated failure time (AFT) model, 165
Access to RWD, 12–15
Activation functions, *158*
Adaptive Pathways, 1, 9, 18
Age-adjusted incidence rate (AAIR), 49–50, 60, *60*
Akaike information criterion (AIC), 93
Alexin Pharmaceuticals, Inc., 73
AlphaFold, 154
Alternative/innovative payment models, 120
Amazon Web Services (AWS), 168–169
American Cancer Society, 58
American Society of Clinical Oncology (ASCO)
Net Health Benefit Score, **118**
Annual Report to the Nation on the Status of Cancer, 55
Artificial intelligence (AI), 151–155
building of, 152–153
definition of, 152
in drug development, 153–155
reasons for, 151
Association of the British Pharmaceutical Industry (ABPI), 30
Average annual percentage change (AAPC), 55

B

Baseline covariate selection and checking, 93–96, *95*, **96**
Batten disease, Brineura® for, 76–82, **77**, **79–82**
Bayesian information criterion (BIC), 93

Bayesian methods, 101–114
meta-analysis of drug safety data, 107–113, **110–112**
sensitivity analysis of unobserved confounder, 102–107, **104–106**
Bipartite matching, 133–134
Birth defects, spermicide effect on, 104–106, **104–106**
Blincyto® label expansion, for minimal residual disease positive acute lymphoblastic leukemia, 85–87
Brineura®, for Batten disease, 76–82, **77**, **79–82**
Brodalumab, suicidal risk of, 108–110
Burden of disease, 121

C

Causal inference, with real-world data, 129–132
Centers for Disease Control and Prevention (CDC), 48
Central processing unit (CPU), 153
Clinical development, external control using RWE and historical data in, 71–98
baseline covariate selection and checking, 93–96, *95*, **96**
comparability of data, 89–90
comparison across trials, for label expansion, 83–87, **85**
objectively study design, 98
propensity score method, 90–93
prospectively plan, 98
sensitivity analysis, 96–98, *97*
single-arm trial, 72–83
comparability of endpoints between active arm and historical control arm, 76–82, **77**, **79–82**
objective endpoint and higher treatment effect, 73–76, **74–76**
supportive evidence, 82–83, **83**
study design, 87–89

Printed in the United States
By Bookmasters